Veterinary Parasitology

The Practical Veterinarian

Veterinary Neurology
Shawn P. Messonnier, ISBN 0-7506-7203-X

Veterinary Anesthesia
Janyce L. Cornick-Seahorn, ISBN 0-7506-7227-7

Veterinary Parasitology
Lora Rickard Ballweber, 0-7506-7261-7

Coming Soon

Veterinary Toxicology
Joseph D. Roder, ISBN 0-7506-7240-4

Veterinary Dermatology
Karen A. Moriello, ISBN 0-7506-7299-4

Veterinary Oncology
Kevin A. Hahn, ISBN 0-7506-7296-X

Small Animal Dentistry
Paul Q. Mitchell, ISBN 0-7506-7321-4

Veterinary Parasitology

Lora Rickard Ballweber, D.V.M., M.S.

Associate Professor of Veterinary Medicine,
College of Veterinary Medicine, Mississippi State University,
Mississippi State

Series Editor
Shawn P. Messonnier, D.V.M.
Paws & Claws Animal Hospital, Plano, Texas

BUTTERWORTH
HEINEMANN

Boston   Oxford   Auckland
Johannesburg   Melbourne   New Delhi

Every effort has been made to ensure that the drug dosage schedules within this text are accurate and conform to standards accepted at time of publication. However, as treatment recommendations vary in the light of continuing research and clinical experience, the reader is advised to verify drug dosage schedules herein with information found on product information sheets. This is especially true in cases of new or infrequently used drugs.

 Recognizing the importance of preserving what has been written, Butterworth–Heinemann prints its books on acid-free paper whenever possible.

 Butterworth–Heinemann supports the efforts of American Forests and the Global ReLeaf program in its campaign for the betterment of trees, forests, and our environment.

Library of Congress Cataloging-in-Publication Data
Ballweber, Lora Rickard, 1958–
    Veterinary parasitology / Lora Rickard Ballweber.
        p. ; cm. — (Practical veterinarian)
    Includes bibliographical references and index.
    ISBN 0-7506-7261-7 (alk. paper)
        1. Veterinary parasitology. I. Title. II. Series.
    [DNLM: 1. Parasitic Diseases, Animal—Handbooks. SF 810.A3 B193v 2001]
    SF810.A3 B35 2001]
    636.089'696—dc21   00-063083

British Library Cataloguing-in-Publication Data
A catalogue record for this book is available from the British Library.

The publisher offers special discounts on bulk orders of this book.
For information, please contact:

Manager of Special Sales
Butterworth–Heinemann
225 Wildwood Avenue
Woburn, MA 01801-2041
Tel: 781-904-2500
Fax: 781-904-2620

For information on all Butterworth–Heinemann publications available, contact our World Wide Web home page at: http://www.bh.com

10 9 8 7 6 5 4 3 2 1

Printed in the United States of America

Contents

Series Preface

The Practical Veterinarian series was developed to help veterinary students, veterinarians, and veterinary technicians find answers to common questions quickly. Unlike larger textbooks, which are filled with detailed information and meant to serve as reference books, all the books in The Practical Veterinarian series are designed to cut to the heart of the subject matter. Not meant to replace the reference texts, the guides in our series complement the larger books by serving as an introduction to each topic for those learning the subject matter for the first time or as a quick review for those who already have mastered the basics of each subject.

The titles for the books in our series are selected to provide information for the most common subjects one would encounter in veterinary school and veterinary practice. The authors are experienced and established clinicians who can present the subject matter in an easy-to-understand format. This helps both the first-time student of the subject and the seasoned practitioner to assess information often difficult to comprehend.

It is our hope that the books in The Practical Veterinarian series will meet the needs of readers and serve as a constant source of practical and important information. We welcome comments and suggestions that will help us improve future editions of the books in this series.

Shawn P. Messonnier, D.V.M.

Preface

Unknowingly, I was first exposed to the discipline of veterinary parasitology as a youngster when my grandfather, Roy V. Stambaugh, gave me his copy of a 1923 USDA publication on the diseases of horses. In thumbing through it, I came upon an illustration of bots that were living in the stomach of the horse. While repulsed, I was at the same time fascinated that such a lifestyle was occurring with apparently little harm to the horse! Perhaps that is why, years later, I chose to accept an assistantship to study for a Master's in parasitology rather than ruminant nutrition, and I have thoroughly enjoyed veterinary parasitology over essentially the past 20 years. As first a student and now a veterinary medical educator, I have seen numerous reference materials on this subject. Many texts have become standards in the required book list, but the most common complaint from veterinary students is they are not user-friendly and are too verbose. Therefore, I was delighted to have the opportunity to write a text that I hope is user-friendly. The outline format was chosen because it is designed to present information in a succinct, easy-to-read, and readily accessible format, thus, making this a quick reference guide to the nuts and bolts of the parasites of veterinary importance designed for the veterinary medical student.

When designing this book, I was confronted with the same question we are all confronted with in our courses: what material to include. The first decision was whether to limit it to the usual dogs, cats, horses, etc., or to include birds, reptiles, rodents, and other small mammals. Shear volume of material made the choice for me—it would have to be limited to traditional domesticated animals (including poultry) with a few rodents and small mammals included in the arthropod section. Next was which actual parasites to include. Decisions here were governed by whether the parasite is common, has dire consequences if missed, or possesses some unique attribute or ability. Some parasites are encountered so infrequently that inclusion in a quick reference guide is not feasible. Others, such as *Spirocerca lupi*, are included because of a unique attribute; in this case, its association with neoplasia. Still others, such as *Acanthocheilonema* (=*Dipetalonema*) *reconditum*, are included because of the difficulty in differentiating diagnostic stages from those of other, more pathogenic parasites; in this case, distinguishing microfilariae from those produced by the heartworm, *Dirofilaria immitis*. Although some parasites near and dear to me were not included, I believe that those essential to a veterinary medical education are.

The book begins with an introduction explaining some basic concepts of parasitology and taxonomic classification. Chapter 2 is devoted solely to ectoparasites. Chapter 3 is an introductory chapter to the endoparasites, describing the characteristics and generalized life cycles of each group (protozoans, nematodes, cestodes, digenetic trematodes, acanthocephalans). Host-parasite lists are provided here as well. The subsequent chapters describe the parasites according to body organ system. Chapters 4 to 6 describe the parasites of the gastrointestinal tract, Chapter 7 describes the cardiopulmonary system, and Chapter 8 covers the remaining organ systems. Geographic distribution and relative significance to both veterinary medicine and public health are included for each parasite as a guide to the student as to the general importance of the parasite.

Information related to treatment of helminths has been summarized in tables for approved compounds available in the United States. Dosages and treatment schedules should be verified on package inserts prior to use. In cases where approved drugs are not available, information on types and dosages of drugs used successfully is included within the text. However, the reader is reminded that this constitutes extra-label drug use and it is the responsibility of the attending veterinarian to determine the dosage and best treatment for the animal. Always be aware of contraindications; for example, many collies and dogs of related herding breeds may suffer potentially fatal idiosyncratic reactions to ivermectin at doses as low as 100 mg/kg.

I would like to acknowledge Dr. Robert Bergstrom who offered me that assistantship in veterinary parasitology those many years ago and fostered my fascination with this subject. I would also like to thank Dr. Eric Hoberg and past and present colleagues at Mississippi State University, including Drs. Carla Siefker, Alan Rathwell, Harry Jacobson, George Hurst, Carolyn Boyle, Sharon Black, Terry Engelken, and Linda Pote, for their help and stimulating discussions over the past few years. Finally, I express sincere appreciation to my husband for his patience and understanding when I needed to be working rather than fishing, and to the rest of my family who do not know exactly what it is I do, but have always supported my decision to do it.

L.R.B.

Veterinary Parasitology

1

Introduction

Symbiosis refers to any association, either temporary or permanent, that exists between two organisms of different species. There are several types of symbiotic relationships, including predator-prey, phoresis, mutualism, commensalism, and parasitism. In the *predator-prey* relationship, the association is one that is very short and results in harm (i.e., death) to one member while benefiting the other. *Phoresis* refers to a relationship in which one member of the association is mechanically carried about by the second member with no harm inflicted on either. *Mutualism* refers to a relationship in which both members of the association benefit as a result of the relationship. *Commensalism* refers to a relationship in which one member of the association benefits while the second member receives neither benefit nor harm. Finally, *parasitism* refers to a relationship in which one member of the association—the parasite—lives in or on the second—the host. The parasite derives nutritional benefit from the host and is usually considered harmful to the host, although the degree of harm can vary greatly. It is the parasites and parasitic diseases of domestic animals that we refer to as the discipline of veterinary parasitology, the subject of this book.

To understand parasites and the diseases they cause, one must first understand what a species is and the concepts of classification. Although not perfect, the most widely accepted definition of a species is an interbreeding population that is reproductively isolated from other such populations. For example, horses are host to many species of small strongyles. As many as 15–20 species of these parasites may be found living in the colon of the same horse at the same time, yet they cannot interbreed and are, thus, separate species. We recognize the fact that many of these species are related, some more closely than others, by considering them to be in the same genus or in closely related genera within the same family. These relationships, then, are the basis of the Linnaean system of classification. There are millions of organisms on earth, each of which may have a different common name in different regions of the world. Conversely, the same common name may be used in different regions of the world to refer to different species. In order to bring about stability and universality, a system of classification has been devised in which all organisms are given a Latin binomial. This consists of a genus name (capitalized) followed by the species name (lowercase). Both genus and species names are italicized. Each species refers to a specific organism and both genus and species names are given when referring to that particular organism, for example, *Dirofilaria immitis* for the heartworm of dogs. Similar species are grouped within the same genus, similar genera within the same family, similar families within the same order, similar orders within the same class, similar classes within the same phylum, and similar phyla grouped together in the same kingdom. In order to communicate with colleagues, it is important to at least learn the species names of the parasites.

Identification is the process of determining to which of these taxonomic groups an organism belongs. It is, generally, based on morphologic characteristics that are used to describe a certain species, genus, family, etc. *Diagnosis*, on the other hand, usually refers to the process of determining the cause of a disease. In this book, the term *diagnosis* is used to refer to the process of determining the presence of or how to identify a particular parasite species and not the determination of the cause of the clinical signs present. For example, diarrhea in a young calf may have a bacterial or viral cause and have little or nothing to do with the coccidial infection present. However, identification of oocysts in the feces may lead the uninitiated to misdiagnose coccidiosis. Always remember—**infection does not equal disease.**

2

Arthropods

Ectoparasites, most of which are arthropods, are those parasites that live on the body of the host. Some spend their entire life on the host, others spend only parts of their life on the host, while still others only occasionally visit the host. The ectoparasites most veterinarians deal with directly are those that live all or much of their life on the host. Those that are periodic visitors to the host are not usually on the animals when presented to the practitioner. Although called upon to treat the effects of these periodic parasites, most veterinarians are not directly involved in their control. Consequently, this chapter focuses on those parasites spending all or much of their life on the host with only brief mention of the periodic parasites.

Classification of the Arthropods

Kingdom: Animalia

Phylum: Arthropoda

Class: Arachnida (scorpions, spiders, mites, and ticks)

Order: Acarina (mites and ticks)

Class: Insecta (insects)

Order: Mallophaga (chewing or biting lice)

Anoplura (sucking lice)

Siphonaptera (fleas)

Diptera (two-winged flies)

Importance

- Intermediate hosts for various parasites.
- Vectors for bacteria, viruses, and other pathogens.
- Direct causal agents of disease.
- Produce venoms that may be toxic.

Morphology

- Arachnids: body divided into two parts (cephalothorax [fusion of head and thorax] and abdomen) or completely fused; adults with four pairs of legs; antennae absent; wingless.

- Insects: body divided into three parts (head, thorax, abdomen); adults with three pairs of legs; antennae present; wings present or absent.

Ticks (Arachnida)

Ticks are divided into two families: the Argasidae (soft ticks) and the Ixodidae (hard ticks). Table 2–1 outlines the important characteristics of each family.

Life Cycle

- Simple metamorphosis with larval and nymphal stages resembling adults.
- Separate sexes with females laying eggs off the host.
- Larva (six legs, no reproductive organs) hatches, feeds on host and molts to nymph.
- Nymph (eight legs, no functional reproductive organs) feeds on host and molts to another nymph (soft ticks) or adult (hard ticks).
- Soft ticks have two or more nymphal stages; hard ticks have only one.
- All adult hard ticks feed on blood whereas not all adult soft ticks do.
- Soft ticks tend to live inside (burrows, dens, hutches, etc.), feed rapidly, and spend relatively little time on the host. Hard ticks tend to live outdoors, feed slowly, and spend longer time on the host.

Table 2–1 Important Characteristics of Soft and Hard Ticks

Character	Argasidae (Soft Ticks)	Ixodidae (Hard Ticks)
Scutum	Absent	Present • males—covers entire dorsal surface • females—covers part of dorsal surface
Mouthparts	Hidden when viewed from the dorsal surface	Visible when viewed from the dorsal surface
Feeding	Larvae feed slowly, over several days; nymphs and adults feed quickly, several times	Larvae, nymphs, and adults feed once, requiring several days to repletion
Life stages	Egg, larva, two or more nymphs, adult	Egg, larva, nymph, adult

- Most ticks cannot tolerate direct sunlight, dryness, or excessive rainfall; tick activity decreases during the cold months and increases during spring, summer, and fall.

- Hard ticks can be classified as either one-host (all stages on one host), two-host (two stages on one host), or three-host (all stages on different hosts) ticks.

Common Soft Ticks in North America

ARGAS SPP.

- In the United States, distributed along the Gulf of Mexico and the Mexican border.

- Parasitize wild and domestic birds, occasionally humans.

- Active primarily in evening hours.

- Annoyance leads to decreased egg production; heavy infestations may cause anemia.

- Development from egg to adult may take as little as 30 days; may survive months (larvae, nymphs) or more than 2 years (adults) without a blood meal.

OTOBIUS MEGNINI (SPINOSE EAR TICK)

- Generally distributed throughout North America.

- Parasitize cattle, horses, other domestic animals, and humans.

- One-host tick in which larvae and nymphs feed in the ear canal; unfed nymphs can survive as long as 2 months.

- Adults have vestigial mouthparts and do not feed; therefore, adult females lay a single clutch of eggs.

Common Hard Ticks in North America

RHIPICEPHALUS SANGUINEUS (BROWN DOG TICK)

- Three-host tick with all stages preferring dogs; can feed on humans.

- Originally found in the tropics; cannot overwinter in cold, temperate regions but will survive indoors in these areas; found in most of the United States and parts of southeast Canada.

- Egg to egg development may be completed in as little as 2 months; unfed adults may survive for over a year.

- Transmit *Babesia canis, Erlichia canis,* possibly *Hepatozoon americanum.*

AMBLYOMMA SPP.

- Two species are common—*Amblyomma americanum* (lone star tick) and *Amblyomma maculatum* (Gulf coast tick).

- Both are three-host ticks—adults prefer feeding on larger animals (cattle and other livestock) and other stages prefer feeding on foxes and similar-sized animals.

- In the United States, *A. maculatum* is distributed along Atlantic and Gulf coastal areas, whereas *A. americanum* is distributed in the southeastern region, into the Midwest and on the Atlantic coast.

- *Ambylomma americanum* can produce severe anemia and may transmit tularemia, Rocky Mountain spotted fever, and Lyme disease.

- *Amblyomma maculatum* produces painful bite wounds that swell and may become secondarily infected; implicated as a cause of tick paralysis; transmit *Hepatozoon americanum.*

DERMACENTOR SPP.

- *Dermacentor variabilis* (American dog tick)—disjunct populations occur across the United States, into Canada, and Mexico.

- *Dermacentor andersoni* (Rocky Mountain wood tick)—widely distributed across western United States and Canada.

- Both are three-host ticks—larvae and nymphs prefer feeding on small rodents, adults prefer larger animals (including dogs and humans).

- Both can transmit Rocky Mountain spotted fever, tularemia, and can cause tick paralysis.

IXODES SPP.

- Several species or subspecies found across the United States.

- Three-host tick with larvae and nymphs preferring small rodents and adults preferring deer.

- Transmits Lyme disease.

Other Important Genera

BOOPHILUS SPP.

- Two species of importance in North America— *Boophilus microplus* and *Boophilus annulatus* (American cattle tick).

- One-host ticks with *B. annulatus* preferring cattle and *B. microplus* preferring large animals in general (cattle, goats, deer, etc.).

- Has been eradicated from the United States and, therefore, if encountered must be reported to state and federal authorities.

- *Boophilus annulatus* transmits Texas cattle fever (*Babesia bigemina*); both can transmit *Anaplasma marginale*.

HAEMAPHYSALIS SPP.

- Important parasite of wild mammals and birds; rarely of dogs, cats, or humans.

- Three-host ticks distributed from Alaska to Argentina.

Diagnosis

Ticks should be collected carefully in order to keep the mouthparts intact. Preserving intact specimens in 70% ethanol or isopropyl alcohol is recommended, although 5% formalin will do. The specific identification of ticks can be challenging, particularly if dealing with larval or nymphal forms. However, adults can be identified to genus using the shape of their capitulum and length of their mouthparts, the presence or absence of markings on the scutum, and body structures. Table 2–2 presents key morphologic characteristics that can be used to distinguish the North American genera of hard ticks.

Treatment and Control

For dogs, dichlorvos, carbaryl, fipronil, and selamectin can be used. Fipronil on cats is highly effective. Flea and tick collars are available for dogs and cats. To control *R. sanguineus* indoors, spray building with Diazinon. Remove vegetation and debris from bed and yards to decrease tick survival. Spray or dust with acaricide to kill those that remain.

For lactating dairy cattle, coumaphos and dichlorvos can be used. These and malathion may be used in non-lactating beef and dairy cattle. Coumaphos is effective for horses. Environmental modification for livestock is often impractical.

Insecticidal dusts or emulsion concentrates are used in the treatment of *O. megnini* infestations.

Table 2–2 Key Morphologic Characteristics Used to Distinguish the North American Genera of Hard Ticks and *Boophilus*

Genus	Anal Groove*	Basis Capituli or Mouthparts	Eyes	Scutal Markings	Festoons
Ixodes	Anterior	Mouthparts long	Absent	Inornate†	Absent
Rhipicephalus	Posterior	Hexagonal basis capituli	Present	Inornate	Present
Amblyomma	Posterior	Mouthparts much longer than basis capituli	Present	Ornate	Present
Dermacentor	Absent	Rectangular basis capituli	Present	Ornate	Present
Haema-physalis	Posterior	Second palpal segment flared laterally	Absent	Inornate	Present
Boophilus	Absent	Hexagonal basis capituli, short mouthparts	Present	Inornate	Absent

*Location of groove, if present, in relation to anus.
†Inornate = no white marks on the scutum; ornate = white marks present on scutum.

Mites (Arachnida)

Mites can be divided into two major groups: sarcoptiform and nonsarcoptiform mites. The sarcoptiform mites can be subdivided into those that burrow or tunnel within the epidermis and those that do not. Sarcoptiform mites are distinguished from nonsarcoptiform mites by possessing a round to oval-shaped body. The legs of sarcoptiform mites also have pedicels (stalks) at the tips that may be long or short. If long, they may be jointed or unjointed. Suckers may be present at the tip of the stalk. These characteristics are very important for identification. Although geographic distribution varies with species of mite, in general, mites are found throughout the world.

Life Cycle

- Simple metamorphosis with larval and nymphal stages resembling adults.
- Separate sexes with females laying eggs on the host.
- Larva (six legs) hatches, may or may not feed, and molts to nymph.
- Nymph (eight legs) feeds on host and molts to another nymph (sarcoptiform mites living on surface) or adult (burrowing sarcoptiform mites; nonsarcoptiform mites).
- Except for some mites of birds, mites tend to spend entire life on the host; for most mites, transmission

is primarily by direct contact although fomites can play a role.

Sarcoptiform Mites

TUNNELING SARCOPTIFORM MITES Table 2–3 presents the host spectrum and characteristic lesions of the common tunneling sarcoptiform mites.

SURFACE-DWELLING SARCOPTIFORM MITES Table 2–4 presents the host spectrum and characteristic lesions of the common surface-dwelling sarcoptiform mites.

Non-Sarcoptiform Mites

***DEMODEX* SPP.** These host-specific mites live in the hair follicles and sebaceous glands of humans and most domestic animals. In most animals, these mites are considered normal, nonpathogenic fauna of the skin. However, particularly in the dog, serious disease can result. Transmission is by direct contact. The cigar-shaped body makes these mites easily recognizable.

Demodex canis
- Localized demodecosis: patchy alopecia, especially of the muzzle, face, and bony projections on extremities; nonpruritic; most recover spontaneously; recurrence is rare.

Table 2-3 Host, Species, Key Characteristics, and Lesions Caused by Tunneling Sarcoptiform Mites

Mite	Host	Lesions	Common Sites	Other
Sarcoptes scabei v. canis	Dogs	Initially erythematous, then papular; becoming crusty, thickened with alopecia, pruritis	Ears, lateral elbows, ventral abdomen	Zoonotic
Sarcoptes scabei v. suis	Pigs	Inflammation, erythema, alopecia, with intense pruritis	Head (ears, nose, eyes) initially; spreads to neck, shoulders, back	Zoonotic

(continues)

Table 2-3 *(Continued)*

Mite	Host	Lesions	Common Sites	Other
Notoedres cati	Cats Rabbits	Yellow crusts, thickened skin, alopecia	Starts on ears; spreads to face, neck, paws, and hindquarters	Most common cause of feline scabies
Trixacarus caviae	Guinea pigs	Dry, scaly skin with alopecia, dermatitis, extreme pruritis	Back, neck, shoulders	Infestations can lead to anorexia and death
Cnemidocoptes mutans	Poultry Wild birds	Hyperkeratosis with legs becoming thickened, deformed	Legs	Common name: scaly leg

Cnemidocoptes pilae C. jamaicensis	Parakeets Canaries	Leg lesions as for C. mutans; crusty mass on beak	Shanks and pads of feet, cere, vent area, back	Common name for facial lesions = scaly face
Cnemidocoptes gallinae	Poultry Pigeons	Inflammation, pruritis; feathers break easily	Back, top of wing, breast, thighs, vent area	Birds may actively pull out feathers

Table 2-4 Host, Species, Key Characteristics, and Lesions Caused by Surface-Dwelling Sarcoptiform Mites

Mite	Host	Lesions	Common Sites	Other
Psoroptes cuniculi	Rabbits	Dried crust in pinna; brown discharge; otitis media may result	Ears	Can also be found on horses, goats, sheep
Psoroptes bovis	Cattle	Pruritic areas consisting of papules, crusts, thickened skin	Withers, back, rump	Reportable and quarantinable
Psoroptes ovis	Sheep	Extremely pruritic; constant rubbing leads to self-mutilation; wool falls out; skin	Wooled areas of the body	Has been eradicated from the United States

Chorioptes spp.	Ruminants Horses	becomes thickened, cracks, bleeds easily; sheep become debilitated and can die	Skin of lower hind legs, tailhead, escutcheon	Reportable in some states
Otodectes cyanotis	Dogs Cats Ferrets	Intensely pruritic; much dark cerumen produced; head shaking can cause hematoma of the aural pinna	External ear, ear canal; has been found around the base of the tail	If untreated, perforation of the tympanic membrane can occur

- Generalized demodecosis: occurs as a result of an immunodeficiency; diffuse alopecia, erythema, and secondary bacterial infections; pruritic; rancid odor; difficult to ameliorate; poor prognosis.

Other Species These species are usually nonpathogenic; however, lesions have been associated with infestations. As for the dog, concomitant diseases are usually present with severe infestations.

- *Demodex cati* and *D. gatoi* (cat) can cause alopecia, erythema, scaly or crusty dermatitis on face, neck, and ears.

- *Demodex bovis* (cattle) and *D. caprae* (goats) can cause pinhead and larger-sized pustules; found on the shoulders, trunk, and lateral aspect of the neck.

- *Demodex ovis* (sheep) can cause localized, scaly lesions; rare.

- *Demodex phylloides* (pigs) can cause pustules around the eyes and on the snout; can spread to ventral surface of the body.

- *Demodex caballi* and *D. equi* (horses) may produce pruritis, alopecia with scaling, or pustules; starts on the neck or withers, spreading to head, forelimbs, and back.

- *Demodex aurati* and *D. criceti* (hamsters, gerbils) can cause alopecia with scaling or scabs; found on the rump and back (hamster) or face (gerbil).

PNEUMONYSSOIDES (=PNEUMONYSSUS) CANINUM

- Oval, pale yellow; 1.0–1.5 mm in length; all legs are on the anterior half of the body.

- Lives in nasal and paranasal sinuses of dogs; prevalence in the United States is unknown.

- Generally thought to be nonpathogenic; has been associated with sneezing, sinusitis, labored breathing, and disorders of the central nervous system (a result of the sinusitis).

CHEYLETIELLA SPP.

- Species include *Cheyletiella blakei* (cats), *C. parasitivorax* (rabbits), and *C. yasguri* (dogs).

- Up to 386 × 266 μm in size; have large hook-like accessory palpi on anterior end.

- Mites are very motile; resemble moving flakes of dandruff (common name: walking dandruff).

- Causes a dry, scaly dermatitis; mild alopecia; perhaps skin thickening.

- May infest humans causing a mild dermatitis.

DERMANYSSUS GALLINAE (RED MITE OF POULTRY) AND ORNITHONYSSUS SYLVIARUM (NORTHERN FOWL MITE)

- Morphologically similar; approximately 1 mm in length.

- Parasitize chickens, wild birds; occasionally humans.

- *Ornithonyssus sylviarum* usually found on birds, but also can be found in nests and poultry houses; *D. gallinae* usually found off birds.

- Feeding activities cause irritation, weight loss, decreased egg production, and anemia; may lead to death.

Diagnosis

The experienced clinician often can make an accurate diagnosis based on the typical distribution and manner of the spread of lesions. However, a positive diagnosis depends on recovery and identification of the mites. Skin scrapings, deep enough to draw blood, are the most common diagnostic tool. Some mites are extremely difficult to find; therefore, negative skin scrapings are inconclusive and animals should be examined repeatedly. Scrapings should be at the margins of active lesions. Additionally, for *Demodex* spp., areas of normal skin should be scraped to determine if the infection is generalized. For *Cnemidocoptes* spp., remove and examine the underside of a loose scale. A strong hand lens may be used to view *Cheyletiella* on the animal.

Table 2–5 presents a key to differentiate the common sarcoptiform mites. Characteristic morphologic features of nonsarcoptiform mites have already been presented.

Treatment and Control

Dogs and cats: oral or SQ ivermectin at 0.2–0.4 mg per kg or topical ivermectin at 0.5 mg per kg is effective against sarcoptic mange in dogs. Clip hair and remove crusty material with keratolytic shampoo first. Ivermectin at 0.3 mg per kg and doramectin at approximately 0.3 mg per kg has been effective against notoedric mange in cats. Otodectic acariasis in dogs and cats requires a thorough cleaning of the ear canal followed by acaricidal otic solutions. Selamectin is approved for use against this parasite. Oral (three treatments at weekly intervals) or SC (two treatments at 2 weeks apart) ivermectin at 0.2–0.4 µg per kg is effective in dogs. Ivermectin at 0.2–0.5 µg per kg administered orally, SC, or topically is effective in cats. Treatment intervals for oral and SC in cats is as for dogs; use a minimum of two treatments given 2 weeks apart for pour-on. For demodectic mange in dogs, the localized form has been treated with 1% rotenone

Table 2–5 Key to the Genera of Common Sarcoptiform Mites

1a. Short, unjointed pedicels.	2
1b. Long pedicels	3
2a. Pedicels on first, second, and fourth pairs of legs of females and all legs of males; body of males with large, posterior lobes.	*Chorioptes*
2b. Pedicels on first and second pairs of legs of females and all legs of males; body of male with small, posterior lobes.	*Otodectes*
3a. Long, jointed pedicels	*Psoroptes*
3b. Long, unjointed pedicels	4
4a. Anus at posterior margin of body	*Sarcoptes*
4b. Anus on dorsal surface of body	*Notoedres*

ointment or 5% benzoyl peroxide once or twice daily. Do not use Amitraz for treatment of the localized form. However, Amitraz is approved and recommended for use against the generalized form. Continue treatment until no live mites are found on two successive skin scrapes. Daily oral ivermectin at 0.6 mg per kg until resolution of infection (4 months) and daily oral milbemycin oxime at 0.52–3.8 mg per kg for varying periods has also been used with mixed success. For *P. caninum*, milbemycin oxime at 0.5–1.0 mg per kg orally once a week for 3 weeks was effective. For *Cheyletiella*, acaricidal shampoos approved for use on dogs or cats are effective as is fipronil in dogs. Ivermectin at 0.2–0.4 mg per kg every 7 (orally) or 14 (SQ) days for 6–8 weeks or pour-on ivermectin at 0.5 mg per kg given 2 weeks apart has also been used. Be sure to treat premises with residual acaricidal spray.

Ruminants: acaricides effective against lice are also good for chorioptic mange in cattle. Eprinomectin is approved for use in lactating dairy cattle. Sarcoptic mange is reportable in cattle; should it occur, treatment and control requirements will be outlined at that time. Psoroptic mange is also reportable and treatment and control requirements will be outlined at that time.

Horses: lindane applied two times at weekly intervals has been effective. Thoroughly clean stall and associated equipment (e.g., feed buckets, curry combs).

Pigs: ivermectin at 0.3 mg per kg SQ is used against sarcoptic mange.

Birds: efforts against *D. gallinae* are directed towards the environment. Periodic removal of litter and nest materials, thorough cleaning, and high-pressure application of residual acaricides are recommended. For control of *O. sylviarum*, spray birds with appropriate ectoparasiticide such as malathion, carbaryl, or permethrin. As with all medications, read and follow label directions. Cnemidocoptic mites may be treated with ivermectin at 0.2 mg per kg, administered parenterally or orally.

Guinea pigs: *T. caviae* can be treated with two doses of ivermectin at 0.2–0.5 mg per kg SQ or orally, given 1 week apart.

Rabbits: *P. cuniculi* can be treated with two injections of ivermectin at 0.2–0.4 mg per kg given 2 weeks apart.

Lice (Insecta)

Lice are distributed across two orders, the Anoplura (sucking lice) and the Mallophaga (biting or chewing lice). Table 2–6 outlines the important characteristics of each family. Although geographic distribution varies according to each species of louse, in general, lice are distributed worldwide.

Life Cycle

- Simple metamorphosis with nymphal stages resembling adults.

- Spend entire life on the host; transmission primarily by direct contact, but fomites can also play a role.

- Separate sexes with adult females laying small (0.5–1.0 mm), whitish, oval eggs (nits); attached firmly to hair or feathers.

Table 2–6 Important Characteristics Distinguishing the Two Orders of Lice

Character	Anoplura (Sucking Lice)	Mallophaga (Chewing Lice)
Color	Tend to be gray or red depending on how much blood has been ingested	Tend to be yellow
Mouthparts	Piercing mouthparts	Chewing mouthparts
Head	Somewhat pointed, narrower than thorax	Rounded head, broader than thorax
Life stages	Egg, three nymphs, adult	Egg, three nymphs, adult
Attachment	Tends to remain attached to animal	Tends to be mobile, easy to remove

- Nymphs hatch from eggs; three nymphal stages occur prior to reaching the adult stage.
- After mating, the adult female will lay eggs and the life cycle begins again.
- The time from egg to egg can take as little as 3–4 weeks.
- Eggs generally do not hatch and neither nymphs nor adults will live much longer than 1 week if removed from the host.

Common Lice

- Lice are relatively host specific with most species of animals having some type of louse (common species and hosts are presented in Table 2–7); human lice (*Phthirus pubis, Pediculus humanus*) can occasionally be found on dogs.
- Sucking lice do not parasitize cats or birds.

Importance

- Most lice problems manifest under crowded conditions, often in winter.
- The presence of either type of louse can cause irritation, pruritis, scratching, licking, and restlessness leading to loss of condition, poor weight gain, decreased milk production, etc.
- Sucking lice can cause anemia.
- Bite wounds can become secondarily infected.

Table 2-7 Common Species of Chewing (Order: Mallophaga) and Sucking (Order: Anoplura) Lice Associated with Domestic Animals

Host	Chewing Louse	Sucking Louse
Birds	*Menopon* spp. (poultry) *Gonoides* spp. (poultry) *Columbicola* spp. (pigeons)	None
Cats	*Felicola subrostratus*	None
Dogs	*Trichodectes canis*	*Linognathus setosus*
Swine	None	*Haematopinus suis*
Sheep	*Damalinia (=Bovicola) ovis*	*Linognathus pedalis* (also goats) *Linognathus ovillus* (also goats)
Goats	*Damalinia (=Bovicola) caprae* *Damalinia (=Bovicola) limbata*	*Linognathus stenopsis* *Linognathus africanis*
Horses	*Damalinia (=Bovicola) equi*	*Haematopinus asini*
Cattle	*Damalinia (=Bovicola) bovis*	*Haematopinus eurysternus* *Linognathus vituli* *Solenopotes capillatus*
Rats/mice	None	*Polyplax spinulosa/Polyplax serrata*
Guinea pigs	*Gliricola porcelli* *Gyropus ovalis*	None
Gerbils	None	*Hoplopleura meridionidis*

- *Trichodectes canis* is an intermediate host of *Dipylidium caninum*; *Linognathus setosus* is an intermediate host for *Acanthocheilonema reconditum*; *Haematopinus suis* transmits swine pox and probably *Eperythrozoon*.

Diagnosis

Lice and their eggs can be detected through careful examination of hair or feathers and are easily seen with the naked eye. A hand-held magnifying lens may assist in their visualization.

Treatment and Control

Dogs and cats: carbaryl shampoos, sprays, or dips, applied in two treatments at 1 week intervals, are effective.

Beef and nonlactating dairy cattle: numerous sprays, dips, and pour-ons are available for use against lice as are insecticidal ear-tags. Macrolide injectibles and pour-ons have excellent activity against anopluran infestations and pour-ons also work against mallophagans. If a herd has a history of infestation, fall treatment is recommended to avoid winter increase in lice populations. Beware of potential host-parasite reactions to cattle grubs that may be concurrently in the esophagus or spinal canal (see *Hypoderma*).

Lactating dairy cattle: a few compounds that can be applied as sprays or used in back rubbers or dust bags are available for this group of animals. Eprinomectin is also approved and has no withdrawal time.

Pigs: injectible or premix formulations of avermectins or pour-on organophosphates are available for lice control.

Horses: two spray applications of coumaphos 2 weeks apart are effective. Dusting horses with a mixture of rotenone and a synergized pyrethrin in winter may be less stressful.

Fleas (Insecta)

Adult fleas are wingless, laterally compressed insects with powerful hind legs allowing them to jump great distances. They have piercing-sucking mouthparts that enable them to feed on a host's blood by piercing a blood vessel and imbibing the blood from the lumen.

Life Cycle

- Complex metamorphosis with egg, maggot-like larval stages, pupa, and adults.

- Adults are parasitic; other stages are found primarily in the host's environment.

- Separate sexes with adult females laying small (about 0.5 mm long), oval eggs on the host or in the environment.

- Larvae hatch from eggs; three larval stages growing from about 2 mm to 5 mm in size, white, turning brown after feeding (primarily on flea feces).

- Third larval stage pupates; pupal stage is stage most resistant to environmental stress and chemical control efforts.

- Heat, carbon dioxide, and movement stimulate adults to emerge from pupae.
- Fleas tend to survive best in humid conditions.

Fleas Encountered in North America

CTENOCEPHALIDES FELIS **AND** *CTENOCEPHALIDES CANIS*

- Parasitize a wide variety of mammals; will feed on humans.
- *Ctenocephalides felis* is the most commonly encountered flea of cats and dogs.
- Generally distributed throughout the United States, particularly prevalent in humid areas.
- Life cycle can take as little as 3 weeks or as long as 20 months.
- Feeding causes irritation resulting in the animal biting and scratching; can cause anemia in very heavy infestations.
- Some animals become sensitized to the salivary secretions resulting in an intensely pruritic reaction (flea-bite hypersensitivity or flea allergy dermatitis).
- Intermediate host for *Dipylidium caninum, Acanthocheilonema reconditum;* transmits *Bartonella henselae* (cat scratch fever).

ECHIDNOPHAGA GALLINACEA **(STICKTIGHT FLEA)**

- Parasitize poultry and other domestic birds; will feed on dogs, cats, rabbits, horses, and humans.

- Present in United States as far north as Kansas and Virginia.
- Life cycle completed in 30–60 days.
- Females remain attached at site of feeding; causes swelling and ulceration; if near eyes, lesions may cause blindness.

XENOPSYLLA CHEOPIS (ORIENTAL OR TROPICAL RAT FLEA)
- Parasitize rats; will feed on humans.
- Present in United States as far north as the northernmost states.
- Life cycle completed in as little as 3 weeks.
- Primary importance is as vector of plague (*Yersinia pestis*).

PULEX IRRITANS (HUMAN FLEA)
- Parasitize humans; will feed on dogs, cats, pigs, and rats.
- Life cycle takes about 1 month to complete.
- This is a human parasite capable of transmitting plague; when recovered from a pet, must tactfully explain to the owners they are the reason the animal has fleas.

Treatment and Control

Dogs and cats: lufenuron, fipronil, and imidacloprid have dramatically changed flea control. All can be administered at monthly intervals although lufenuron also has a long-acting injectible formulation providing action longer than a 1-month duration. Lufenuron does not kill adult fleas, but prevents eggs from hatching. Because the vast majority of all fleas are found in the environment as eggs, larvae, or pupae, environmental control should be considered in flea control programs with these or any other products. Numerous over-the-counter products are available as shampoos, collars, or topicals, which provide adequate control when combined with proper environmental control programs.

Myiasis-Producing Flies (Insecta)

The larvae of certain dipterans are capable of developing in the tissues of many domestic animals. This results in a condition called myiasis. There are two types of myiases: (1) facultative myiasis—larvae are free-living, but can become parasitic under certain conditions; and (2) obligatory myiasis—larvae are always parasitic, i.e., without a proper host, the flies cannot complete their life cycle.

Life Cycle

- Complex metamorphosis with egg, larval stages (instars), pupa, and adults.
- Separate sexes with adult females laying eggs or larvae on host or in environment.
- Larvae hatch from eggs; three larval stages (maggots).

- Third larval stage pupates with adults emerging from pupae.

Obligatory Myiasis-Producing Flies

Adults of the obligatory myiasis-producing flies tend to resemble honeybees. They have only vestigial mouthparts and, therefore, do not feed. They are quite annoying to their hosts as the females buzz around the animal, laying her eggs. These flies are extremely host- and site-specific. Because they are so specific, the third-stage larvae can be provisionally identified to genus based on host and site alone. However, first- and second-stage larvae must be differentiated from larvae of the facultative myiasis-producing flies, particularly if in an abnormal host.

OESTRUS OVIS (SHEEP NASAL BOT)
- Females fly around nostrils of sheep and goats during the hottest part of the day; deposit tiny, white to yellow, first-stage larvae; crawl into nasal sinuses, and develop into large (3 cm), dark brown third-stage larvae.
- Third-stage larvae crawl out of the nostrils or are sneezed out; pupate in the ground; adults emerge 3–6 weeks later; if begin pupating in fall, pupate overwinter and adults emerge in spring; larvae can also overwinter in nares of host.
- Larvae produce a purulent rhinitis or sinusitis leading to head shaking, restlessness, snorting; may lead to damage of cribriform plate and subsequent brain injury.

- Diagnosis based on seeing large, dark brown larvae dropping out of nostrils; postmortem diagnosis achieved by sawing skull in half longitudinally, rinsing key areas with water, and examining the rinsings for larvae with a magnifying lens.
- Ocular myiasis of humans has been reported.

GASTEROPHILUS (OR *GASTROPHILUS*) SPP. (HORSE STOMACH BOT)

- Three species in horses—*G. nasalis*, *G. hemorrhoidalis*, *G. intestinalis*.
- Adult females attach elongate, operculated eggs to hairs of the intermandibular space (*G. nasalis*), the lips (*G. hemorrhoidalis*), or forelegs and shoulders (*G. intestinalis*) during late summer and early fall.
- Eggs around the mouth hatch spontaneously; those elsewhere hatch in response to sudden warmth provided by the breath of the horse.
- Larvae penetrate and migrate in oral mucosa and tongue; eventually reach the stomach or duodenum and attach to the wall.
- Third-stage larvae pass out in feces in spring; pupate in the soil for 3–9 weeks.
- Generally considered benign parasites except for the annoyance associated with the adults; mucosal and submucosal inflammation and mucosal ulceration of the duodenum has been associated with infections of *G. nasalis* in ponies.

- Diagnosis is based on seeing eggs attached to hairs or distinctive third-stage larvae in feces; one can also find larvae at necropsy; usual attachment sites are the first ampulla of the duodenum for *G. nasalis*, the nonglandular part of the stomach at the margo plicatus or in the saccus cecus for *G. intestinalis*, the duodenum and rectum for *G. hemorrhoidalis*.

HYPODERMA SPP. (CATTLE GRUBS; HEEL FLIES)

- Two species infesting cattle and bison—*H. bovis* (northern cattle grub), *H. lineatum* (common or southern cattle grub).

- *Hypoderma lineatum* is present in the southern United States; both species are present in the northern United States and into Canada.

- Entire life cycle of both species takes about 1 year to complete.

- Adult *H. lineatum* becomes active with the start of warm weather, remaining active for about 2 months; *H. bovis* becomes active about the time *H. lineatum* stops, remaining active into summer.

- Larvae hatch spontaneously, crawl down hair shaft, penetrate skin, and migrate through the subcutaneous tissues.

- Larvae, in 4–5 months, come to rest in either the submucosal connective tissue of the esophagus (*H. lineatum*) or the epidural fat (*H. bovis*); remain there for about 3 months.

- Resume migration to subcutaneous tissues of the back, cut breathing holes and increase in size as they develop to the third-stage larvae.

- When fully developed, larvae exit through breathing holes, fall to ground, and pupate with adult flies emerging in 4–5 weeks.

- Egg-laying activity disturbs animals; they run about aimlessly (gadding) in an attempt to escape the flies; results in loss of production.

- Larval infestation leads to carcass damage and damage to hide from the breathing holes; if animals are treated when larvae are in resting sites (esophagus, spinal canal), signs of bloat/choke or central nervous system disease can result.

- Diagnosis is made by finding either the eggs on hairs of the legs or the larvae in the back.

- Infestations of horses and humans have been reported, although rare.

COCHLIOMYIA HOMINOVORAX (AMERICAN PRIMARY SCREWWORM)

- Only fly in North America attracted to uncontaminated skin wounds of domestic animals; will infest any living warm-blooded animal (including humans) with a wound.

- Adult females lay many eggs in batches of 15–400 at the edge of wounds.

- Larvae hatch spontaneously and enter wound feeding on secretions and living flesh; become third-stage larvae in 5–7 days.

- Larvae drop to ground, burrow in soil and pupate; adults emerge in one to several weeks.

- Life cycle can be completed in as little as 24 days; larvae cannot overwinter where soil freezes.

- Fatal if not treated; can kill a full-grown steer in 5–7 days.

- Massive eradication efforts used insecticidal treatment of all infested animals and release of sterile flies to eliminate this parasite from the United States and Mexico. Because females mate once and the wild population of the fly is relatively small, release of billions of sterile males swamps the population and significantly reduces the chance of a successful mating.

- Occasionally reenters the United States in imported animals; larvae encountered in wounds (particularly of imported animals or animals in border areas with Mexico) must be differentiated from facultative myiasis-producing flies. If encountered, it must be reported to state and federal authorities.

CUTEREBRA SPP.
- Primarily parasites of rabbits and rodents; will infest dogs and cats; although rare, most frequent cause of endemic human myiasis in North America.

- Adult females lay eggs near entrances to burrows or along rabbit runs.

- Larvae hatch in response to presence of animal, crawl into fur, and enter subcutaneous tissues of host through natural body openings.

- Cut breathing holes and develop to large (up to 3 cm), black third-stage larvae in subcutaneous cysts.

- In dogs and cats, generally found in neck and head region in late summer and early fall; also found in aberrant sites including anterior chamber of the eye and the brain.

- Generally benign unless secondary bacterial infection of cyst occurs or larvae migrate to aberrant sites.

- Diagnosis is based on finding characteristic cysts with breathing holes in which second- or third-stage larvae are usually present.

Facultative Myiasis-Producing Flies

GENERA OR SPECIES INVOLVED

- *Lucilia* (green or copper bottle flies)
- *Phoenicia* (green bottle flies)
- *Phormia* (black blow flies)
- *Calliphora* (blue bottle flies)
- *Sarcophaga* (flesh flies)
- *Cochliomyia macellaria* (secondary screwworm)

IMPORTANCE

- Normally, adults lay eggs in carrion or feces; also attracted by suppurative wounds, necrotic areas, skin soiled with urine, feces, or vomitus (bacterial growth generates odors attractive to flies); condition called fly strike or strike.

- Females feed and lay eggs; larvae hatch; feed on necrotic debris and exudates.

- Larvae can cause further damage; some may invade healthy subcutaneous tissue producing large cavities or tunnels; host becomes anorexic and weak.

- Infestation can lead to death as a result of septicemia, toxemia, or shock.

DIAGNOSIS Diagnosis of maggot infestation is not difficult because the larvae are easily observed in the wound or within the hair coat. Species diagnosis, however, is dependent on morphologic characteristics of the larvae, particularly of the spiracular plates on the posterior end of the larvae. Depending on the situation, larvae may need to be differentiated from those of *Cochliomyia hominivorax*. In that case, collect larvae, preserve in 70% ethanol, and submit to proper authorities for identification.

Treatment and Control

For bots of sheep, horses, and grubs of cattle, avermectins are effective. Treatment of cattle should be done immediately after fly season ends but before the larvae reach the esophagus or spinal cord; destruction of larvae in these tissues causes severe inflammatory reactions and clinical signs corresponding to the locality of the larvae. The danger period for treatment is estimated to be 6–8 weeks before the larvae appear in the back, which occurs around mid-September in the southern United States, late December in areas such as Ohio, and late January in the more northern areas of the United States. Although adverse reactions are considered to be rare occurrences these days, they must still be kept in mind in designing parasite control programs for cattle.

Infestations of *C. hominivorax* are reportable; should it occur, treatment and control requirements will be outlined at that time.

Treatment of *Cuterebra* consists of manual extraction of the larva.

Treatment of facultative myiasis infestations includes debriding area, applying appropriate insecticides, and, if present, treating secondary bacterial infections.

Keds (Insecta)

This is a group of dorso-ventrally flattened insects that may or may not have wings. Although there are numerous species of keds in North America, only one is generally encountered in veterinary medicine.

Melophagus ovinus (Sheep Ked)

- Entire life cycle spent on sheep or goats; transmission is by direct contact although fed females may live up to a week off the host.

- No eggs present on host; larvae retained in abdomen until ready to pupate; time until adult emergence depends on ambient temperature.

- Most numerous in cold months (fall, winter) with fewer present during warm months; more prevalent in northern United States and Canada.

- Feed on blood which may cause anemia; bites are also pruritic leading to biting, scratching, and rubbing which damages wool; ked feces stains wool, decreasing value.

- Coumaphos, malathion, and other insecticides are effective against this parasite.

Biting Gnats and Mosquitoes (Insecta)

These dipteran insects are periodic parasites; that is, the only role vertebrate hosts have in the insects' life cycle is as a food source for the adult females. However, these insects have a primary role as biological vectors of various disease-causing agents. Because the insects are only periodic parasites, they are usually not found on the animals.

Life Cycle

- Complex metamorphosis with egg, up to five larval stages, pupa, and adults.

- Separate sexes with adult females laying eggs in aquatic or semi-aquatic habitats.

- Larvae hatch from eggs; final larval stage pupates; adults emerge.
- Adult females need bloodmeal for egg development; males do not feed on blood.

Simulium *spp. (Black Flies; Buffalo Gnats)*

- Tiny flies (1–6 mm long) that tend to swarm; require well-aerated water for eggs; limits geographic distribution to areas of swiftly running water.
- Serrated, scissor-like mouthparts; lacerates tissue to form a pool of blood; bites very painful; ears, neck, and abdomen are favored feeding sites.
- Swarming and biting can cause annoyance, resulting in decreased production in livestock.
- Transmit *Leucocytozoon* spp. (hemoparasites of birds), *Onchocerca gutterosa.*

Culicoides *spp. (No-See-Ums, Biting Midges)*

- Tiny gnats (1–3 mm long); habitat requirements vary with species; strong fliers that tend to remain close to breeding grounds; active at dusk or dawn.
- Bites are very painful; favored feeding sites are either on dorsal or ventral aspect of host, depending on species involved.
- Bites cause annoyance.

- Allergic dermatitis in horses; begins as discrete papules on dorsum; areas of alopecia form as hair mats, crusts, then falls off; intensely pruritic leading to scratching and rolling behavior which may lead to injury or secondary infection.

- Transmit bluetongue virus, *Onchocerca cervicalis, Haemoproteus,* and *Leucocytozoon* spp. (hemoparasites of birds).

Anopheles *spp.,* Aedes *spp.,* Culex *spp.* (Mosquitoes)

- Small flies (3–6 mm long) that tend to swarm; lay eggs on water or in dry places that flood periodically; complete entire life cycle in as little as 1–2 weeks.

- Have piercing-sucking mouthparts; pierces blood vessel and feeds from the lumen; bites can be painful.

- Swarming and biting can cause annoyance leading to decreased production in livestock; rarely causes anemia.

- Transmit eastern and western equine encephalitis, *Plasmodium* species (malaria), *Dirofilaria immitis.*

Treatment and Control

Because these pests are not found on the host except when feeding, insecticidal treatment is ineffective unless repeated every few days; this becomes too expensive and impractical. Consequently, control is aimed at killing pre-adult stages.

Horse Flies, Deer Flies (Insecta)

Like mosquitoes and biting gnats, horse flies and deer flies are periodic parasites in which only the adult females feed on blood.

Life Cycle

- Complex metamorphosis with egg, larval stages, pupa, and adults.
- Separate sexes with adult females laying eggs in aquatic or semi-aquatic habitats.
- Larvae hatch from eggs, drop into the water or mud; first- and second-stage larvae do not feed; later stages feed on insect larvae, snails, young frogs, organic matter, etc.; in temperate regions, larvae may over-winter and pupate the following spring.
- Pupae are found in dry soil; adults are active only during warmer months in temperate regions.
- Adult females need blood for egg development; interrupted feeders—feeds several times in multiple sites on one or more hosts until replete; preferred feeding sites are ventral abdomen, legs, neck, withers; prefers feeding on larger animals.

Genera Involved

- *Tabanus* (horse flies)
- *Chrysops* (deer flies)

Importance

- Large flies (up to 3.5 cm with horse flies being bigger than deer flies).

- Bite very painful; scissor-like mouthparts lacerate tissue to form pool of blood; bite causes restlessness, annoyance, avoidance behavior, which interferes with grazing and resting resulting in decreased production.

- Mechanical vectors of anaplasmosis, anthrax, equine infectious anemia virus.

- *Tabanus* spp. are intermediate hosts for *Elaeophora schneideri* (arterial worm of deer, elk, sheep).

Treatment and Control

Difficult to kill or repel. Flies rarely enter roofed areas so stabling during hours of peak fly activity helps. Keeping animals inside a fence 2.4 m in height with a 0.6 cm mesh helps reduce the attack rate. Keep grazing animals away from the edge of wooded areas also helps reduce the attack rate.

Stable Flies, Horn Flies, Face Flies (Insecta)

These flies are periodic parasites with different feeding habits. Both male and female stable and horn flies feed on blood whereas only female face flies feed on mucus, saliva, and tears.

Life Cycle

- Complex metamorphosis with eggs, larvae, pupae, and adults.

- Separate sexes with adult females laying eggs in decaying organic matter (stable fly) or fresh cow manure (horn fly, face fly).

- Larvae hatch from eggs; final larval stage pupates; adults emerge.

Stomoxys calcitrans *(Stable Fly)*

- Flies similar in size to house fly (6–7 mm long); piercing-sucking mouthparts.

- Distributed primarily in central and southeastern United States.

- Horse preferred host, but will feed on most domestic animals and humans; feed 1–2 times per day depending on ambient temperature; feed primarily on legs and flanks of cattle and horses, ears of dogs, ankles of humans.

- Bites are painful; annoyance can lead to decreased production in livestock.

- Mechanical vectors of anthrax and equine infectious anemia virus; intermediate host for *Habronema microstoma* (stomach nematode of horses).

Haematobia irritans *(Horn Fly)*

- Dark-colored, small flies (3–6 mm long); piercing-sucking mouthparts.
- Distributed throughout North America.
- Feed on cattle; rarely on horses, sheep, dogs.
- Adults spend most of life on host, leaving only to lay eggs; adults cluster on shoulders, back, and sides; if ambient temperature < 70°F, cluster around base of horns; if quite hot, cluster on ventral abdomen.
- Irritation associated with feeding activities results in lost beef and/or dairy production; of all blood-sucking flies in the United States, this fly is most responsible for reduced weight gains and milk production.
- Intermediate host for *Stephanofilaria stilesi* (filarid nematode of cattle).
- Can cause a focal, midline dermatitis in horses.

Musca autumnalis *(Face Fly)*

- Medium-sized flies (about 6 mm long); sponging mouthparts.
- Generally distributed in North America except for the southwestern United States; adults will hibernate in large groups inside buildings.
- Feed on all types of livestock, horses, and bison.
- Flies' feeding activity is irritating to the host; can lead to decreased production.

- Mechanical vectors of infectious keratoconjunctivitis (pinkeye).

- Intermediate host for *Thelazia* spp. (eyeworms) of cattle.

Treatment and Control

Treatment with insecticides is possible; read the label and follow directions carefully. Insecticidal ear tags can be effective fly control aids. Pour-on avermectins are effective against horn flies

3

Introduction to the Endoparasites

Endoparasites are those parasites that live within the body of the host. There are four major groups of endoparasites—nematodes, acanthocephalans, platyhelminths (trematodes and cestodes), and protozoans. Table 3–1 provides distinguishing characteristics of the helminthic parasites.

Nematodes

Appearance and Morphology

- Variable length, 1 mm to several meters.
- Body covered with cuticle, may form specialized structures (e.g., alae).
- Usually sexually dimorphic with males smaller than females.

Table 3–1 Characteristics of the Major Helminth Groups

| Characteristic | Phylum | | | |
| | Nemathelminthes | Acanthocephala | Platyhelminthes | |
			Cestodes	Trematodes
Body shape	Round, elongate, generally tapering at both ends, not segmented	Round, elongate, anterior with spiny proboscis, appears to be segmented	Dorso-ventrally flattened, elongate, segmented	Dorso-ventrally flattened, leaf-shaped, not segmented
Coelem	Pseudocoel	Pseudocoel	Acoelomate	Acoelomate
Digestive tract	Complete (mouth, esophagus, intestine, anus)	Absent	Absent	Incomplete (mouth, esophagus, intestine)
Sexes	Dioecious (separate sexes)	Dioecious	Monoecious (hermaphroditic)	Monoecious (exceptions)

Classification

Nematodes are divided among two classes: the Secernentea and the Adenophorea. The Adenophorea contains the whipworms, capillarids, and *Trichinella spiralis*, while the Secernentea contains the remainder of the parasitic nematodes. Numerous advancements have been made in our understanding of the relationships of many of these parasites. As a consequence, some nematodes have been reassigned to different genera (Table 3–2). While some consider presenting current and future veterinarians with proper taxonomic nomenclature to be impractical, others consider not to do so to be a disservice to their continuing education and development. Therefore, those changes in species level nomenclature which have achieved general acceptance among the scientific community are presented herein. Tables 3–3, 3–4, 3–5, 3–6, and 3–7 present the orders, families, and species of the parasitic nematodes by host group.

Life Cycle

- All nematodes, whether parasitic or free-living, have the same stages in the life cycle: egg, four larval stages (L_1 molts to L_2 molts to L_3 molts to L_4), immature adult (sometimes called L_5), which matures into adult.

- Stages occurring in the external environment are subjected to stresses (temperature, desiccation, sunlight, etc.) that may kill or delay development (develop-

Table 3–2 Reclassification of Some Parasites Important to Veterinary Medicine

Old Name	New Name	Intermediate/ Paratenic Host	Definitive Host	Site of Infection
Capillaria aerophila	*Eucoleus aerophila*	Earthworm	Canids, felids, mustelids	Lungs
Capillaria böhmi	*Eucoleus böhmi*	None known	Fox, dog	Nasal, paranasal sinuses
Capillaria plica	*Pearsonema plica*	Earthworm	Canids, mustelids	Urinary bladder
Capillaria feliscati	*Pearsonema feliscati*	Earthworm	Felids	Urinary bladder
Capillaria putorii	*Aonchotheca putorii*	Earthworm	Mustelids, raccoon, pig, cat	Stomach, small intestine
Capillaria bovis	*Aonchotheca bovis*	None known	Cattle	Small intestine

Capillaria annulatus	*Eucoleus annulatus*	Earthworm	Chickens, wild game birds	Esophagus, crop
Capillaria contortus	*Eucoleus contortus*	None or earthworm	Wide variety of birds	Esophagus, crop, mouth
Capillaria obsignata	*Baruscapillaria obsignata*	None	Wide variety of birds	Small intestine
Dipetalonema reconditum	*Acantho-cheilonema reconditum*	Fleas, lice	Canids	Subcutaneous tissues
Toxocara cati	*Toxocara mystax*	Rodents	Felids	Small intestine
Ostertagia circumcincta	*Teladorsagia circumcincta*	None	Ruminants, especially sheep	Abomasum
Babesia equi	*Theileria equi*	Ixodid ticks	Horses	Red blood cells

Table 3–3 Classification of Nematodes Encountered in Pigs

Class	Order	Family	Species
Secernentea	Rhabditida	Strongyloididae	*Strongyloides ransomi*
	Strongylida	Trichostrongylidae	*Hyostrongylus rubidus*
		Strongylidae	*Oesophagostomum dentatum; O. brevicadum*
		Syngamidae	*Stephanurus dentatus*
		Metastrongylidae	*Metastrongylus apri; M. pudendodectus; M. salmi*
	Ascaridida	Ascarididae	*Ascaris suum*
	Spirurida	Spirocercidae	*Ascarops strongylina*
			Physocephalus sexalatus
Adenophorea	Enoplida	Trichuridae	*Trichuris suis*
		Trichinellidae	*Trichinella spiralis*

Table 3-4 Classification of Nematodes Encountered in Horses

Order	Family	Species
Rhabditida	Strongyloididae	*Strongyloides westeri* *Halicephalobus* *(=Micronema) deletrix** *Rhabditis (=Pelodera)* *strongyloides**
Strongylida	Dictyocaulidae	*Dictyocaulus arnfieldi*
	Trichostrongylidae	*Trichostrongylus axei*
	Strongylidae	*Strongylus vulgaris; S.* *edentatus; S. equinus* *Cyathostomum* spp. and other small strongyles
Ascaridida	Ascarididae	*Parascaris equorum*
Oxyurata	Oxyuridae	*Oxyuris equi*
Spirurida	Habronematidae	*Draschia megastoma* *Habronema muscae;* *H. microstoma*
	Thelaziidae	*Thelazia lacrymalis*
	Onchocercidae	*Onchocerca cervicalis*

*Not mentioned further in this book.

Table 3–5 Classification of Nematodes Encountered in Ruminants

Class	Order	Family	Species
Secernenta	Rhabditida	Strongyloididae	Strongyloides papillosus
	Strongylida	Trichostrongylidae	Ostertagia ostertagia;*
			Teladorsagia circumcincta
			Trichostrongylus axei;
			T. colubriformis
			Haemonchus contortus;
			H. placei
			Cooperia spp.
		Molineidae	Nematodirus spp.
		Strongylidae	Oesophagostomum radiatum; O. venulosum; O. columbianum
			Chabertia ovina
		Ancylostomatidae	Bunostomum phlebotomum

	Dictyocaulidae	*Dictyocaulus filaria; D. viviparus*
	Protostrongylidae	*Muellerius capillaris Protostrongylus* spp.†
Spirurida	Thelaziidae	*Thelazia skrjabini; T. gulosa*
	Gongylonematidae	*Gongylonema pulchrum; G. verrucosum*†
	Onchocercidae	*Setaria labiatopapillosa Onchocerca gutterosa; O. lienalis*
	Filariidae	*Stephanofilaria stilesi*
	Trichuridae	*Trichuris bovis; T. ovis; T. skrjabini*
Adenophorea Enoplida	Capillariidae	*Aonchotheca bovis*

*Several other species of *Ostertagia* exist and may cause or contribute to disease.

†Not mentioned further in this book.

Table 3–6   Classification of Nematodes Encountered in Dogs and Cats

Class	Order	Family	Species
Secernentea	Rhabditida	Strongyloididae	*Strongyloides stercoralis*
	Strongylida	Ancylostomatidae	*Ancylostoma caninum; A. tubaeforme; A. braziliense*
			Uncinaria stenocephala
		Molineidae	*Ollulanus tricuspis**
		Angiostrongylidae	*Aleurostrongylus abstrusus*
			Angiostrongylus spp.*
		Filaroididae	*Filaroides osleri; F. hirthi**
		Crenosomatidae	*Crenosoma vulpis**
	Ascaridida	Toxocaridae	*Toxocara canis; T. mystax*
		Ascarididae	*Toxascaris leonina*
			Baylisascaris procyonis
	Spirurida	Spirocercidae	*Spirocerca lupi*
		Physalopteridae	*Physaloptera* spp.
		Thelaziidae	*Thelazia californiensis*

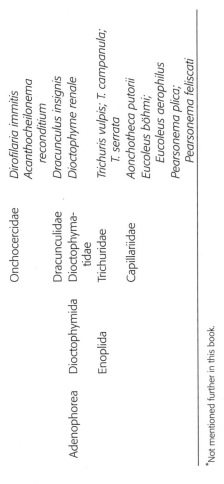

Adenophorea	Dioctophymida	Onchocercidae	*Dirofilaria immitis* *Acanthocheilonema* *reconditium*
		Dracunculidae	*Dracunculus insignis*
		Dioctophyma- tidae	*Dioctophyme renale*
	Enoplida	Trichuridae	*Trichuris vulpis; T. campanula;* *T. serrata*
		Capillariidae	*Aonchotheca putorii* *Eucoleus böhmi;* *Eucoleus aerophilus* *Pearsonema plica;* *Pearsonema feliscati*

*Not mentioned further in this book.

Table 3-7 Classification of Nematodes Encountered in Poultry and Other Gallinaceous Birds

Class	Order	Family	Species
Secernentea	Rhabditida	Strongyloididae	*Strongyloides avium*
	Strongylida	Syngamidae	*Syngamus trachea*
		Heterakidae	*Heterakis gallinarum*
		Ascaridiidae	*Ascaridia galli*
Adenophorea	Enoplida	Capillariidae	*Eucoleus annulatus*
			Eucoleus contortus
			Baruscapillaria obsignata

mental times presented throughout the book are minimum times required under optimal conditions).

- For most parasitic nematodes, the third-stage larva is the infective stage (i.e., the stage that initiates infection in the definitive host); infective larvae cannot feed and are usually ensheathed—the third-stage larvae do not completely shed the cuticular sheath of the second-stage larvae until some point after being ingested; the sheath provides protection against adverse environmental conditions; after the infective L_3 sheds the sheath of the L_2, they are referred to as parasitic L_3.

- Transmission may be direct (no intermediate host required) or indirect (intermediate host required or paratenic host involved).

- Development to adulthood may proceed normally or, under certain circumstances, larvae may arrest development and remain quiescent until reactivated at a later time.

- Adults infect a variety of organs; larval migration may or may not occur depending on species and site of infection.

Acanthocephalans (Thorny-Headed Worms)
Appearance and Morphology

- Variable length, 6 mm to 30+ cm.

- Proboscis is retractable into body; body covered with tegument; absorbs nutrients.

- Usually sexually dimorphic with males smaller than females.

Classification

Higher-level classification of the acanthocephalans is not presented here because only one species, *Macracanthorhynchus hirudinaceus* (swine) has been generally encountered in veterinary medicine. Recognition of the parasite in the host and understanding the characteristics of the phylum are sufficient for most practicing veterinarians.

Life Cycle

- All acanthocephalans have indirect life cycles; stages include egg, acanthor, acanthella, cysticanth, adult.
- Essential first intermediate host is some type of arthropod; simplest life cycle requires only one intermediate host, while more complicated cycles involve the addition of a second or even third intermediate host.
- Adults live in the intestinal tract only; extra-intestinal migration does not occur.

Cestodes
Appearance and Morphology

- Body divided into scolex, neck, strobila.
- Scolex may contain holdfast organs in the form of suckers or slits and/or rostellum armed with hooks.
- Neck is the germinal region from which the strobila arises.

- Strobila is the rest of the body; composed of proglottids each of which contains one set of reproductive organs; proglottids mature as they move away from the neck with gravid (egg-containing) proglottids at end of body.

Classification

The tapeworms of veterinary importance are divided among two groups—the Eucestoda and the Pseudophyllidea. Table 3–8 presents the families and species of these two groups of tapeworms encountered in North America.

Life Cycle

All cestodes have an indirect life cycle; however, the stages vary according to the group involved. Adult tapeworms are found in the intestinal tract (or ducts of associated organs) while larval stages (metacestodes) can be found in a variety of organs.

EUCESTODA

- Stages include egg, hexacanth embryo, metacestode, adult.

- Gravid proglottid usually passes out of host with feces; ruptures releasing eggs.

- Eggs contain embryo with six hooks (hexacanth embryo); must be ingested by intermediate host to develop to metacestode stage.

- Metacestode can take several forms; if ingested by arthropod, develops into cysticercoid; if ingested by mammalian host, develops into cysticercus, strobilocercus,

Table 3–8 Classification of Cestodes Encountered in Veterinary Medicine

Order	Family	Species	Intermediate Hosts	Metacestode Type	Definitive Hosts
Pseudo-phyllidea	Diphyllo-bothriidae	*Diphyllobothrium latum*	Fish	Procercoid, plerocercoid	Dogs
		Spirometra mansonoides		Procercoid, plerocercoid	Dogs, cats
Cyclo-phyllidea	Taeniidae	*Taenia* spp.	Pigs, ruminants, rodents	Cysticercus, coenurus, strobilocercus	Carnivores, humans
		Echinococcus spp.	Ruminants, rodents, humans	Hydatid cyst	Canids, felids
	Anoploceph-alidae	*Anoplocephala* spp.	Mites	Cystercoid	Horses

Avitellinidae	*Moniezia* spp. *Thysansoma actinioides**	Mites Mites	Cystercoid Cystercoid	Ruminants Sheep
Dilepididae	*Dipylidium caninum*	Fleas, lice	Cystercoid	Dogs, cats, humans
Mesocestoididae	*Mesocestoides* spp.*	First IH unknown; Rodents	First metacestode unknown; Tetrathyridium	Canids

*Not mentioned further in this book.

coenurus, hydatid cyst, or tetrathyridium; metacestode type is characteristic of the cestode species involved.

- Definitive host becomes infected by ingesting the infected intermediate host; extra-intestinal migration in the definitive host does not occur.

PSEUDOPHYLLIDEA

- Stages include operculated egg, coracidium (ciliated hexacanth embryo), metacestode, adult.
- Eggs are expelled from the gravid proglottid; pass out with feces.
- Coracidium hatches in water; first intermediate host is a copepod; ingested coracidium develops to procercoid (metacestode).
- Copepod is ingested by the second intermediate host; procercoid develops into another metacestode stage called the plerocercoid.
- Definitive host becomes infected by ingesting the intermediate host containing the plerocercoid; extra-intestinal migration in the definitive host does not occur.

Trematodes

There are two types of trematodes—digenes and monogenes. Monogenetic trematodes have direct life cycles and are primarily ectoparasites of aquatic vertebrates. Digenetic trematodes have indirect life cycles and are endoparasites of a wide variety of vertebrates. Unless the veterinarian is involved in fish farming or treating aquarium fish, monogenetic trematodes are not encountered very often. Consequently, the emphasis of this book will be on the digenetic trematodes.

Appearance and Morphology

- Variable length, 0.5 mm to 10 cm.
- Body is covered with tegument; may have spines.
- Does not have anus; must regurgitate cecal contents to rid body of waste products.
- Most possess a muscular organ of attachment called an acetabulum (ventral sucker).
- Most are hermaphroditic (exception is the schistosomes—blood flukes); self-fertilization or cross-fertilization can occur.

Classification

Table 3–9 presents the families and species of digenetic trematodes encountered in North America.

Life Cycle

- All digenes have indirect life cycles; stages include operculated egg, ciliated embryo (miracidium), asexual reproductive stages (sporocyst, redia), cercaria, metacercaria, adult.

Table 3–9 Classification of the Digenetic Trematodes Encountered in Veterinary Medicine

Family	Species	First Intermediate Host	Second Intermediate Host	Definitive Host
Fasciolidae	*Fasciola hepatica*	Freshwater snails	None	Ruminants, pigs
	Fascioloides magna	Freshwater snails	None	Cervids
Paramphistomatidae	*Paramphisto-mum* spp.*	Freshwater/amphibious snails	None	Ruminants
Dicrocoeliidae	*Dicrocoelium dendriti-cum*	Terrestrial snails	Ants	Cattle
	Platynoso-mum fastosum	Terrestrial snails	Sowbugs/woodlice	Felids

Troglotrematidae	*Eurytrema* spp.*	Terrestrial snails	Probably grasshoppers	Raccoons
	Paragonimus kellicotti	Aquatic/amphibious snails	Crayfish	Dogs, cats, mink, oppossum, raccoon
	Nanophyetes salmincola	Aquatic snails	Numerous fish	Dogs, mink
Diplostomatidae	*Alaria* spp.	Freshwater snails	Tadpoles/frogs	Dogs, cats, wild carnivores

*Not mentioned further in this book.

- First intermediate host is some type of snail; miracidium penetrates or is ingested; asexual reproduction occurs resulting in cercarial stage; one miracidium in can equal hundreds to thousands of cercariae out.

- Cercariae can penetrate and encyst in second intermediate host, encyst on vegetation, or penetrate definitive host (schistosomes); encysted stage is called metacercaria.

- Definitive host becomes infected by ingesting plants or intermediate host with metacercarial stage; the cercariae of blood flukes (schistosomes) are directly infective to the definitive host.

- Juvenile fluke migration can be extensive; adults live in a variety of organs; eggs are passed with the feces.

Protozoa

Protozoans are single-celled organisms, varying greatly in size and shape. Of all the protozoans in the world, only a small number are parasitic. Of these, many are not harmful to the host, although those that are pathogenic can cause severe and devastating disease. The pathogenic parasitic protozoans encountered in veterinary medicine are spread among three major taxonomic groups—Sarcomastigophora (flagellates and amoebae), Ciliophora (ciliates), and Apicomplexa (apicomplexans which include the coccidia). Table 3–10 lists the protozoans that may be encountered in veterinary medicine.

Table 3–10 Parasitic Protozoans Encountered in Veterinary Medicine

Protozoan Group	Species	Host*
Flagellates	*Giardia duodenalis*	Mammals including humans
	Histomonas meleagridis	Gallinaceous birds
	Trichomonas gallinae	Pigeons, chickens, raptors
	Tritrichomonas foetus	Cattle
Ciliates	*Balantidium coli*	Pigs, rats, dogs, primates
Apicomplexans	*Eimeria* spp.	Ruminants, horses, pigs, poultry
	Isospora spp.	Dogs, pigs, cats
	Toxoplasma gondii	Cats, sheep, goats, pigs, humans
	Sarcocystis neurona	Horses, oppossums
	Neospora caninum	Dogs, cattle
	Cryptosporidium parvum	Mammals including humans
	Cryptosporidium andersoni	Cattle
	Cytauxzoon felis	Bobcat, cats
	Babesia bigemina	Cattle
	Babesia caballi	Horses
	Theileria equi	Horses
	Babesia canis	Dogs
	Hepatozoon americanum	Dogs

*Host in which the parasite is most often encountered.

Flagellates

- Possess at least one flagellum for locomotion in the trophozoite stage.
- Reproduce by binary fission.
- Some species form cysts that are resistant to external environmental conditions.

Ciliates

- Possess cilia for locomotion in the trophozoite stage.
- Possess two types of nuclei—macronucleus and micronucleus.
- Form cysts that are resistant to external environmental conditions.

Apicomplexans

- Obligatory intracellular parasites.
- Multiply through strict sequence of asexual and sexual reproduction.
- May have direct or indirect life cycles.

4

Parasites of the Gastrointestinal Tract I—Nematodes

Swine

Stomach

HYOSTRONGYLUS RUBIDUS
- Worldwide distribution in domestic and wild swine; locally significant depending on management and control.
- Common name: red stomach worm of swine.

Life Cycle
- Direct.

- Eggs passed in feces; L_1 develops and hatches; infective L_3 develops in about 1 week.
- Pigs acquire infection by ingesting infective L_3; L_3 enters gastric glands, molts to L_4 then immature adult; returns to lumen and matures to adult.
- Prepatent period approximately 3 weeks.
- Larvae may arrest development in older sows or upon reinfection.

Pathogenesis and Clinical Signs

- Developing larvae can cause blood loss (anemia), acute gastritis with nodule formation.
- Adult worms may be associated with chronic catarrhal gastritis.
- Clinical signs may include decreased feed intake, weight loss or decreased weight gain, diarrhea, and/or agalactia in nursing sows.

Diagnosis

ANTEMORTEM

- Presumptive diagnosis based on finding typical trichostrongyle-type eggs on fecal flotation (Figure 4–1).
- Eggs are oval, thin shelled, $71–78 \times 35–42$ µm, containing morula with 16–32 cells.
- Definitive diagnosis through identification of infective larvae recovered from coproculture (usually not performed by the practitioner).

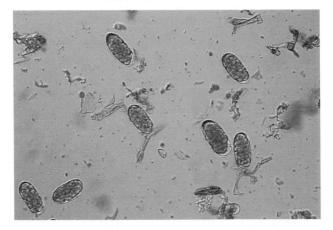

Figure 4–1 Nematode eggs featured here could be either tri-chostrongyle-type or strongyle-type, depending on whether the host was a ruminant, a pig (trichostrongyle-type), or a horse (strongyle-type) (100×).

POSTMORTEM

- Small, red worms, 0.4–1.1 cm in length; may be easily missed on gross necropsy.

Treatment and Control

- See Table 4–1 for anthelmintics.
- Control programs for *Ascaris suum* also control this nematode.

ASCAROPS STRONGYLINA, PHYSOCEPHALUS SEXALATUS

- Worldwide distribution in domestic and wild Suidae; sporadic occurrence.
- Common name: thick stomach worms of swine.

Life Cycle

- Indirect.
- Intermediate host: coprophagous beetles.
- Larvated eggs are passed in the feces; ingested by beetles; L_1 hatches and develops to infective L_3 in approximately 30 days.
- Pigs acquire infection by ingesting beetles containing the infective L_3; larvae mature to adult in stomach.
- Prepatent period is 46–50 days for *A. strongylina* and 30–40 days for *P. sexalatus*.

Table 4–1 Partial List of Nematodical Anthelmintics for Pigs

Active Ingredient	Dosage (mg/kg)	Route	Ascaris	Oesophagostom	Hyostrongylus	Strongyloides	Stephanurus	Metastrongylus	Trichuris
Piperazine[1]	See label	In water	✓	✓					
Pyrantel tartrate	See label	In feed	✓	✓					
Fenbendazole	See label	In feed	✓	✓	✓	✓	✓	✓	✓
Ivermectin[2,3]	0.3	SQ	✓	✓	✓	✓	✓	✓	✓
Doramectin[3]	0.3	IM	✓	✓	✓	✓		✓	
Hygromycin	See label	In feed	✓	✓					✓

[1] Treat at 8–10 weeks of age and repeat monthly or as necessary; treat sows and gilts one month before breeding and again before farrowing.

[2] Also available as a premix that extends spectrum of activity to include *Stephanurus*.

[3] Treat sows and gilts 7–14 days before breeding and again before farrowing; treat feeder pigs upon arrival or prior to moving to clean quarters.

Pathogenesis and Clinical Signs

- Infections may be associated with gastritis.
- Clinical signs may include anorexia, weight loss, or decreased weight gains.

Diagnosis

ANTEMORTEM
- Presumptive diagnosis based on finding eggs on fecal flotation (sodium nitrate probably best medium); eggs similar for both species.
- Eggs are thick-shelled, larvated, 34–40 × 15–20 µm.

POSTMORTEM
- Worms are robust, up to 2.2 cm in length; genera can be differentiated based on morphology of the pharynx.

Treatment and Control

- Drugs effective against *A. suum* should be tried (see Table 4–1).
- Modern intensive management systems have greatly reduced the incidence of these parasites.

Small Intestine

ASCARIS SUUM
- Worldwide distribution in domestic and wild pigs; whether infects humans or not is debated, although

allergic response to eggs has been noted; highly significant.

Life Cycle

- Direct; indirect with paratenic host.

- Eggs passed in feces; infective L_3 develops within the egg in approximately 3 weeks; eggs extremely resistant to environmental conditions, remaining viable up to 5 years.

- Transmission occurs primarily through ingestion of eggs containing infective L_3; undergo hepatic-pulmonary migration—larvae hatch, enter the wall of the small intestine, migrate to the liver, then proceed to the lungs (via caudal vena cava, heart, pulmonary artery, capillaries), and molt to L_4; larvae break out into alveoli and migrate or are coughed up to be swallowed; matures in lumen of small intestine.

- Migratory phase is 10–15 days; prepatent period is 8–9 weeks; live 7–10 months.

- Earthworms and dung beetles can be paratenic hosts.

Pathogenesis and Clinical Signs

- Larvae spend 4–6 days migrating in the liver causing cellular destruction and multiple interstitial hepatitis that will resolve within 3–6 weeks after cessation of larval exposure.

- Pulmonary reactions include petechial and ecchymotic hemorrhages, bronchitis, and edema.

- Adult worms interfere with host nutrition; damage to small intestine is minor, generally limited to a catarrhal enteritis; rarely does obstruction or perforation of the small intestine occur; immune response to repeated exposure causes spontaneous expulsion of adults.

- Clinical signs may include rapid, shallow breathing characterized by audible expiratory efforts (called "thumps") or other signs of severe respiratory distress, unthriftiness, colic, weight loss or reduced weight gain, stunted growth.

- Infections generally more prevalent in young pigs (3–6 months old); older pigs and adults may harbor subclinical infections.

Diagnosis

ANTEMORTEM

- Eggs may be found on fecal flotation.

- Eggs are ovoid, golden brown, thick-shelled with a bumpy appearance, 50–75 × 40–50 µm (Figure 4–2).

- Pigs are coprophagic, therefore, may pass eggs without being infected (false positive).

- Adult worms may be passed in feces (after treatment or spontaneous expulsion).

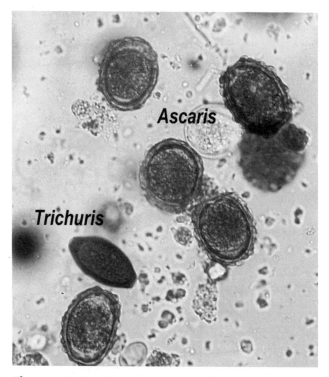

Figure 4–2 Fecal flotation from a pig with both *A. suum* and *T. suis* eggs (200×).

POSTMORTEM

- Adult *A. suum* is the largest nematode occurring in pigs—up to 40 cm in length, very stout, white; found in the small intestine.

- Fibrosis in the liver associated with larval migration appears as white spots (also called "milk spots"); can mince liver or lung and place in Baermann apparatus to recover migrating larvae.

Treatment and Control

- See Table 4–1 for anthelmintics; may need to repeat treatments in 2–3 weeks.

- Strict sanitation must be enforced; treat sows 2 weeks before farrowing; repeat treatment approximately 4 days before farrowing; remove all dirt and fecal contamination from sow by washing and then move to clean farrowing pen; pigs bought for finishing should be treated before entering the unit; further recommendations will depend on the individual producer.

STRONGYLOIDES RANSOMI

- Worldwide distribution; low significance.
- Common name: threadworm.

Life Cycle

- Direct.
- Has two reproductive cycles, a parasitic (homogonic) cycle and a free-living (heterogonic) cycle.

- Only parthenogenetic females are parasitic; eggs are laid in the small intestine and L_1 develops within; larvated eggs are passed with the feces; larvae hatch and develop into either infective L_3 capable of infecting another pig or continue developing to free-living adults; if progress into free-living generation, both males and females develop, mate and produce eggs; offspring of free-living generation are usually parasitic; when environmental conditions are unsatisfactory, the homogonic cycle predominates; when environmental conditions are satisfactory, the heterogonic cycle predominates.

- Routes of transmission to the definitive host include:

    Percutaneous—larvae penetrate the skin, travel by way of blood and lymph to the lungs, migrate up the bronchi to the trachea and are swallowed; mature in the small intestine.

    Peroral—after ingestion of infective L_3, most are thought to penetrate the oral mucosa and migrate as for the percutaneous route; those that are swallowed do not have extra-intestinal migration; rather, they develop directly to parthenogenetic females in the small intestine.

    Transmammary—following percutaneous exposure in older animals, larvae inhibit development during migration in skeletal muscles, subcutis, etc.; shortly after birth, larvae "reactivate" and migrate to the mammary gland and are ingested by nursing piglets; extra-intestinal migration does not occur.

Prenatal—larvae "reactivate" from tissues and migrate to fetus in utero.

- Prepatent period is approximately 4 days after prenatal or transmammary infection and 7–10 days for the other routes; infections tend to peak at 2–3 weeks of age, disappearing at 5–6 weeks.

Pathogenesis and Clinical Signs

- Infection in older animals is usually inapparent and usually so in young animals as well; disease, when it does occur, is present only in young animals.

- Transmammary infection common, although percutaneous also may occur; areas of skin may become erythematous and pustules may be present; catarrhal enteritis may occur; clinical signs may include bloody diarrhea, anemia, severe weight loss.

Diagnosis

ANTEMORTEM

- Eggs may be found on fecal flotation; even though *S. ransomi* eggs are smaller, must use fresh feces to avoid confusion with larvated trichostrongyle-type eggs.

- Eggs are thin-shelled, oval, 45–55 × 26–35 μm, each containing a fully developed larva.

POSTMORTEM

- Adult worms are embedded in the mucosa of the small intestine; worms are extremely small in size (up to 4.5 mm in length) and will be missed at necropsy unless mucosal scrapings are examined under a microscope.

Treatment and Control

- See Table 4–1 for anthelmintics.
- Maintain clean and dry pigpens—larvae cannot survive 5 minutes of drying or 1–2 hours of direct sunlight; treat infected sow 2 weeks prior to farrowing to prevent transmammary transmission.

Cecum and Large Intestine

OESOPHAGOSTOMUM SPP.

- Includes *Oesophagostomum dentatum* and *O. quadrispinulatum.*
- Worldwide distribution in domestic and wild swine; moderate significance, especially in warm and humid regions.
- Common name: nodular worm.

Life Cycle

- Direct.
- Eggs passed in feces; L_1 hatches; develops to infective L_3 within 5 days.

- Pigs acquire infection by ingestion of infective L_3; L_3 migrates into the wall of the cecum or colon; develops and molts to L_4 within the wall; then returns to lumen, molts again, and matures to adult.

- In older animals or on reinfection, larvae may arrest development within the gut wall.

- Prepatent period is 17–21 days; if larvae arrest development, the prepatent period is greatly lengthened.

Pathogenesis and Clinical Signs

- *Oesophagostomum quadrispinulatum* is considered more pathogenic than *O. dentatum*, producing larger nodules.

- Nodular formation may lead to protein-losing enteropathy and hemorrhagic enteritis.

- Clinical signs may include anorexia, diarrhea, weight loss, or decreased weight gain; death may result, but is rare.

Diagnosis

ANTEMORTEM

- Eggs may be found on fecal flotation.

- Eggs are thin-shelled, oval, 60–80 μm, containing morula with 16–32 cells; may be difficult to differentiate from eggs of *Hyostrongylus*.

- Definitive diagnosis is based on identification of larvae recovered from coproculture (usually not performed by the practitioner).

POSTMORTEM

- Adult worms are white, stout, up to 2.0 cm in length.

- *Oesophagostomum quadrispinulatum* tends to be found in the cecum and proximal colon; *O. dentatum* tends to be found more distally.

- Species can be differentiated based on esophageal structure and the length of the tail of the female.

Treatment and Control

- See Table 4–1 for anthelmintics.

- Treatment of sows before farrowing and between weaning and remating helps reduce environmental contamination; other control measures are as for *A. suum.*

TRICHURIS SUIS

- Worldwide distribution in domestic and wild swine; moderate significance.

- Common name: whipworm.

Life Cycle

- Direct.

- Eggs passed in feces; L_1 develops within egg in approximately 3 weeks; does not hatch; larvated eggs resistant to freezing.

- Pigs acquire infection by ingestion of egg containing infective L_1; larvae hatch in the small intestine, enter mucosal glands of cecum and colon, and undergo four molts to immature adult stage; return to lumen with anterior end embedded in mucosa and mature.

- Prepatent period is 6–7 weeks; live approximately 4–5 months.

Pathogenesis and Clinical Signs

- Severe infections usually occur only in young swine.
- Adults are hematophagous and more pathogenic than larvae; can cause catarrhal enteritis with mucosal necrosis and hemorrhage; may facilitate invasion of the colon by enteric bacteria resulting in mucohemorrhagic colitis.
- Clinical signs may include diarrhea, dehydration, anemia, weight loss.

Diagnosis

ANTEMORTEM
- Typical trichurid-type eggs may be found on fecal flotation (Figures 4–2 and 4–3).
- Eggs have a thick, brown shell with a smooth surface, two polar plugs that are light in color and protrude from the ends, 50–60 × 21–25 µm.

POSTMORTEM
- Adult worms are whip-like in appearance, 3–5 cm in length; found attached to mucosal surface of cecum and colon.

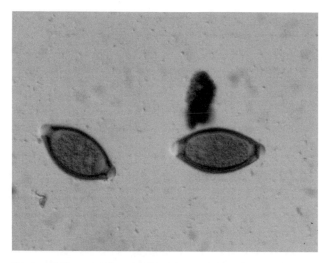

Figure 4–3 Fecal flotation showing typical appearance of whipworm (*Trichuris*) eggs (200×).

Treatment and Control

- See Table 4–1 for anthelmintics.
- Control measures are as for *A. suum.*

Horses

Stomach

DRASCHIA MEGASTOMA, HABRONEMA MUSCAE, H. MICROSTOMA

- Worldwide distribution in horses; sporadic occurrence.

Life Cycle

- Indirect.
- Intermediate hosts = *Musca domestica* (housefly) for *D. megastoma, H. muscae*; *Stomoxys calcitrans* (stable fly) for *H. microstoma.*
- Larvated eggs or hatched L_1 passed in feces, ingested by fly maggot; develops to infective L_3 in fly as pupates.
- Infective L_3 migrate to head of fly, collect in labium; larvae are deposited when fly feeds; if L_3 swallowed by horse or horse ingests infected flies in food or water, larvae enter stomach and mature; if L_3 deposited in cutaneous sores/wounds, maturation and completion of the life cycle do not occur.

- Prepatent period for all three species is approximately 2 months.

Pathogenesis and Clinical Signs

- Stomach infection—adult *Habronema* spp. live on mucosal surface causing mild catarrhal gastritis; adult *D. megastoma* elicit fibrous nodules containing masses of worms and necrotic debris. Clinical signs generally not apparent; nodule formation may cause mechanical interference with pyloric sphincter (rare).

- Cutaneous infection (Summer sores)—caused by larval infection of skin; sites are those areas with open sores or wounds or areas subjected to continuous wetting (e.g., medial canthus of the eye). Characterized by painful, pruritic, nonhealing, granulomatous lesions that protrude above the level of the skin and readily bleed; wart-like lesions on nictitating membrane or skin around the eye can cause corneal abrasion. Lesions do not resolve until winter, after flies become inactive.

Diagnosis

ANTEMORTEM

- Eggs or L_1 difficult to find on fecal flotation; direct fecal smear may be more informative.

- Eggs or L_1 may be found by gastric lavage.

- Eggs of both genera are elongate, thin-shelled, 40–50×10–12 μm.

- Biopsy of cutaneous lesions may show larvae to be present.

POSTMORTEM
- Slender worms, 0.7–2.5 cm in length; found on gastric surface or in nodules.

Treatment and Control

- See Table 4–2 for anthelmintics.
- Fly control or insect repellents to keep intermediate host away.

Small Intestine

PARASCARIS EQUORUM
- Worldwide distribution in horses and donkeys; may be highly significant depending on management and control.

Life Cycle

- Direct.
- Eggs passed in feces; infective L_3 develops within the egg in approximately 2 weeks.
- Transmission occurs through ingestion of eggs containing infective L_3; undergo hepatic-pulmonary migration as for *A. suum.*
- Migratory phase is approximately 3 weeks; prepatent period is 10–12 weeks; may live up to 2 years.

Table 4–2 Partial List of Nematocidal Anthelmintics for Horses

Active Ingredient	Dosage (mg/kg)	Route	Parascaris	Large Strongyles	Small Strongyles	Oxyuris	Habronema	Strongyloides
Piperazine[1]	See label	Oral	✓					
Pyrantel pamoate	6.6	Oral	✓	✓	✓	✓		
Pyrantel tartrate	2.6[2]	In feed	✓	✓	✓	✓		
Oxfendazole	10	Oral	✓	✓	✓	✓		
Oxibendazole	10	Oral	✓	✓	✓	✓		
Fenbendazole	5	Oral	✓[4]	✓	✓	✓		✓[3]
Ivermectin	0.2	Oral	✓	✓	✓	✓	✓	✓
Moxidectin	0.4	Oral	✓	✓	✓	✓	✓	✓

[1]Repeat in 30 days or as needed.
[2]Administered daily.
[3]Dosage of 15 mg/kg required.
[4]Dosage of 10 mg/kg required.

Pathogenesis and Clinical Signs

- Migrating larvae can produce fibrosis in the liver and petechial hemorrhages in the lungs.

- Adults cause a catarrhal enteritis; occasionally, mechanical obstruction of small intestine or bile duct or perforation of small intestine with peritonitis occurs.

- Clinical signs include frequent coughing and bilateral mucopurulent discharge, decreased feed intake, unthriftiness, colic, pot-bellied appearance, diarrhea, death.

- Infections usually more prevalent in suckling and weanling foals; adults may be carriers without apparent clinical signs of infection.

Diagnosis

ANTEMORTEM
- Eggs may be found on fecal flotation.

- Eggs are almost round, golden brown, thick-shelled with a pitted surface, 90–100 μm in size (Figure 4–4).

- Worms may be passed in feces (after treatment or spontaneous expulsion).

POSTMORTEM
- Adult *P. equorum* is the largest nematode occurring in horses—up to 40 cm in length, very stout, white; found in small intestine.

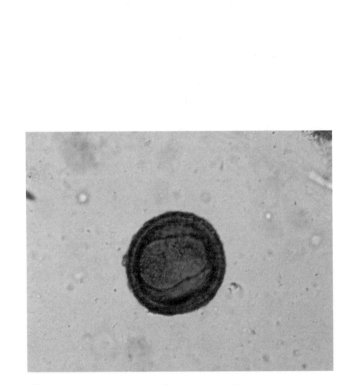

Figure 4–4 Fecal flotation from a horse with *P. equorum* (400×).

Treatment and Control

- See Table 4–2 for anthelmintics.
- Stall sanitation important—ideally, remove manure and bedding and clean with high-pressure cleaner or steam jenney weekly; if too labor intensive, thoroughly clean foaling stall and udder and teats of mare prior to foaling; reliance solely on anthelmintics to decrease environmental contamination may not be effective because the eggs are extremely resistant and tend to accumulate with time.

STRONGYLOIDES WESTERI

- Worldwide distribution in horses and donkeys; low significance.
- Common name: threadworm.

Life Cycle

- Direct.
- Life cycle as for *S. ransomi* except no prenatal transmission; transmammary infection most important route.
- Infections tend to peak at 4–6 weeks of age, disappearing at 20–25 weeks.

Pathogenesis and Clinical Signs

- Infection in older animals inapparent and usually so in young animals as well; disease, when it does occur, is present only in young animals.

- Acute diarrhea most common clinical sign.

Diagnosis

ANTEMORTEM
- Eggs may be found on fecal flotation; even though *S. westeri* eggs are smaller, must use fresh feces to avoid confusion with larvated strongyle-type eggs.
- Eggs are thin-shelled, oval, 40–52 × 32–40 μm, each containing a fully developed larva.

POSTMORTEM
- Adult worms are embedded in the mucosa of the small intestine; worms are extremely small in size (up to 9 mm in length) and will be missed at necropsy unless mucosal scrapings are examined under a microscope.

Treatment and Control

- See Table 4–2 for anthelmintics.
- Keep stall clean and dry.

Cecum and Colon

STRONGYLUS VULGARIS, S. EDENTATUS, AND S. EQUINUS
- Worldwide distribution in horses, donkeys, asses, and zebras; moderate to high significance.

- Common name: large strongyles.
- Mixed infections with small strongyles common.

Life Cycle

- Direct.
- Eggs are passed in feces; L_1 hatches, develops to infective L_3 in approximately 1 week; horses acquire infection by ingestion of infective L_3.
- *Strongylus vulgaris*—larvae penetrate large intestinal mucosa, molt to L_4 by 7 days post-ingestion, then invade the submucosal arterioles; migrate along the intima to cranial mesenteric artery where they molt to immature adults by 3 months post-infection; carried back to intestinal wall within the lumen of the arteries; nodules form around the larvae which eventually enter lumen of the intestine and mature; prepatent period is 6–7 months.
- *Strongylus edentatus*—larvae penetrate intestinal mucosa and migrate to liver via the hepatic portal system; molt to L_4 in liver; after about 8 weeks, migrate back to the subserosa of the gut by way of the hepatic ligaments; nodules form around the larvae where they molt to immature adults; nodules eventually open into the lumen of the large intestine and the parasites mature; prepatent period is approximately 11 months (some authorities state may be as short as 6 months).
- *Strongylus equinus*—larvae penetrate the wall of the large intestine where they molt to L_4 in nodules

formed in the submucosa; larvae leave nodules, enter peritoneal cavity, and migrate to liver; remain within the liver 6–8 weeks, then move to pancreas; molt to immature adults, return to the large intestine, penetrate back to the lumen and mature; prepatent period is approximately 9 months.

Pathogenesis and Clinical Signs

- Adults—usually not considered to be of significance; may cause diarrhea, generalized unthriftiness, anemia.

- Larval *S. edentatus* and *S. equinus* can cause hemorrhagic tracts in the liver and elicit nodule formation in the gut or on the peritoneum; pancreatitis associated with *S. equinus* is rare; clinical signs are not generally present.

- Larval *S. vulgaris* are considered to be the most pathogenic; major pathologic condition is inflammation and thromboses of the cranial mesenteric artery, its branches, and the iliac, celiac, and femoral arteries; may result in aneurysms; thromboembolisms may lodge in smaller vessels of the gut producing ischemic infarctions and ileus of the gut; clinical signs include fever, diarrhea, colic, intermittent or permanent lameness, death.

Diagnosis

ANTEMORTEM

- Can find strongyle-type eggs on fecal flotation (see Figure 4–1).

- Eggs are oval, thin-shelled, grayish in color, 70–90 × 40–50 μm, containing morula with 8–16 cells; eggs of large and small strongyles are very similar and cannot be differentiated, therefore, must be categorized as "strongyle-type" and not specific genus or species.

- Definitive diagnosis of large strongyles can be made on identification of infective larvae recovered from coproculture (usually not performed by the practitioner).

POSTMORTEM

- Adult worms are grayish-red, stout, up to 4 cm in length; found in the cecum and colon; species can be differentiated based on the number and type of tooth-like projections in the buccal cavity.

Treatment and Control

- See Table 4–2 for anthelmintics; resistance to pyrantel has been reported.

- Control programs must be tailored to the individual situation; control should not rely solely on anthelmintics; judicious use of drugs at key times of the year combined with improved pasture management (manual or mechanical removal of feces at least 2 times per week, alternate grazing with ruminants, prolonged destocking of pasture) are key ingredients of an effective control program.

SMALL STRONGYLES OR CYATHOSTOMES

- Worldwide distribution in horses, donkeys, asses, and zebras; moderate to high significance.

- Numerous genera (approximately 13) and species (approximately 40) in North America; multiple species infections and mixed infections with large strongyles common.

Life Cycle

- Direct.

- Eggs are passed in feces; L_1 hatches, develops to infective L_3 in approximately 1 week; horses acquire infection by ingestion of infective L_3.

- Larvae do not undergo extra-intestinal migration; L_3 penetrate the mucosa and submucosa of cecum and colon; molt to L_4, then to adult stage; return to lumen and mature.

- Prepatent period is 4–6 weeks; however, in temperate regions, larvae have a tendency to arrest development prolonging the prepatent period up to 4 months.

- Adult horses primarily responsible for pasture contamination; in temperate regions, eggs hatch and infective larvae tend to accumulate on pasture during late summer and early autumn and sharply decrease over winter; overwintering of eggs partially responsible for pasture contamination in early spring; in subtropical and tropical regions, larvae are present on pasture year round with peaks occurring during the cooler months.

Pathogenesis and Clinical Signs

- Adults may be associated with generalized debilitation or intermittent soft feces.
- Larval presence in mucosa/submucosa stimulates nodule formation; nodules are hemorrhagic (blackish to dark red in color) and contain lymphocytes, plasma cells, and eosinophils.
- Synchronous emergence of arrested larvae can cause a catarrhal or hemorrhagic enteritis and a protein-losing enteropathy as a result of the destruction of cells and disruption of cellular junctions.
- Clinical signs include sudden onset of watery diarrhea, rapid weight loss, emaciation, hypoalbuminemia, colic, death.

Diagnosis

ANTEMORTEM
- Can find strongyle-type eggs on fecal flotation (see Figure 4–1).
- Eggs are oval, thin-shelled, grayish in color, 70–90 × 40–50 μm, containing morula with 8–16 cells; eggs of large and small strongyles are very similar and cannot be differentiated, therefore, must be categorized as "strongyle-type" and not specific genus or species.

- Definitive diagnosis of small strongyles can be made on identification of infective larvae recovered from coproculture (usually not performed by the practitioner).

- Bright red L_4 and immature adults may be passed with the feces or may be observed on gloves after performing rectal palpations.

POSTMORTEM
- Worms are white to dark red, up to 2.5 cm in length; found in the cecum and colon.

Treatment and Control
- See Table 4–2 for anthelmintics; anthelmintic resistance to a variety of compounds is common.

- Essentials of good control programs are as for large strongyles.

OXYURIS EQUI
- Worldwide distribution in horses and donkeys; low significance.

- Common name: pinworm.

Life Cycle
- Direct.

- Adult females migrate to rectum, out anus, and cement masses of eggs on perineal area; infective L_3 develops within the egg in 4–5 days; environmental contamination occurs when cementing fluid dries and cracks allowing eggs to fall off or egg masses are rubbed off by horse's attempt to relieve associated pruritis.

- Horses acquire infection by ingesting eggs containing infective L_3; eggs hatch in the small intestine and larvae move directly to cecum/colon where they mature.

- Prepatent period is 4–5 months.

Pathogenesis and Clinical Signs

- Feeding activities of L_4 may cause inflammation of cecal and colonic mucosa.

- Egg-laying activity of female worms causes pruritis; may lead to persistent rubbing.

- Clinical signs may include vague signs of abdominal discomfort and/or persistent rubbing of tailhead which can lead to broken hairs and "rat tail" appearance or scarification.

Diagnosis

ANTEMORTEM

- Identification of grayish-yellow, scale-like egg masses on the perineal skin.

- Eggs rarely found on routine fecal flotation; detected using "scotch tape" technique—apply a piece of cellophane tape to region, then stick the tape onto a microscope slide and examine for eggs with microscope.

- Eggs are operculated, ovoid, yellowish, thick-shelled, and flattened on one side, may or may not be larvated; 85–95 × 40–45 μm.
- May find gray-white adult females in feces.

POSTMORTEM
- Gray-white, robust worms up to 15 cm in length; mature females with long, pointed tail; found in cecum, colon, and rectum.

Treatment and Control

- See Table 4–2 for anthelmintics.
- Wash, every 4 days, the perineal area and underside of tailhead with soap and water to remove egg masses; make sure feed and water troughs are high enough to prevent fecal contamination.

Ruminants

Abomasum

- Genera include *Haemonchus, Ostertagia, Teladorsagia, Trichostrongylus*; most common worms found in grazing ruminants; worldwide distribution.
- In general, *Ostertagia ostertagi* is the most important nematode among cattle in temperate regions; *Haemonchus contortus* is the most important nematode among sheep and goats; however, mixed

infections with multiple genera occur and usually are responsible for disease.

Haemonchus, Ostertagia, Trichostrongylus, Teladorsagia

Life Cycle

- Direct.
- Basic life cycle essentially the same for these genera; eggs passed in feces; L_1 hatches, develops to infective L_3 in 1–2 weeks; larval development and survival dependent on climate and pasture management—desiccation and direct sunlight are lethal to eggs and larvae.
- Depending on climatic factors, L_3 may overwinter on pasture and be partially responsible for infections the following spring.
- Ruminant acquires infection by ingestion of infective L_3; depending on species, larvae may migrate into gastric glands, then return to the lumen; adult stage reached in 2–3 weeks.
- Prepatent period is 2–4 weeks.
- Some species (*Ostertagia ostertagi* in particular) will arrest development, which significantly alters the prepatent period.

Pathogenesis and Clinical Signs

- Age group most likely to acquire pathogenic numbers of parasites is first year grazing calves, lambs, and kids;

bovine ostertagiosis important in weanling and year-ling classes; poor nutrition and other stress factors may contribute to clinical disease in adult animals.

- Both larval and adult worms may be pathogenic; the clinical picture produced depends on the composition of the parasites present, how many are present, age and nutritional status of the host, and a variety of other factors.

- In mixed infections (the rule rather than the exception), the general pathologic condition is a hyperplastic gastritis and catarrhal enteritis.

- Clinical signs may include diarrhea, rough hair coat, weight loss or decreased weight gain, anemia, inappetence.

- Ostertagiosis in cattle

    Development and emergence of larvae from gastric glands cause cellular destruction; loss of parietal cells causes decreased production of HCl leading to increased abomasal pH; protein digestion ceases when pH is over 4.5–5.0.

    Increased pH also results in loss of bacteriostatic effect and failure to activate pepsinogen to pepsin.

    Cellular destruction results in disruption of junctions leading to enhanced permeability; plasma proteins leak into abomasum resulting in hypoalbuminemia, fluid accumulation in abomasal walls, and peripheral edema (most often manifested as submandibular edema or "bottle jaw").

Lesions consist of single to coalescing, raised, umbilicated nodules in the abomasum; abomasal folds may appear thicker than normal due to edema.

Clinical signs may include diarrhea, dehydration, inappetence, loss of weight or decreased weight gain, death.

Type I ostertagiosis—occurs as a result of recently ingested larvae developing to adulthood without larval inhibition; occurs primarily in young cattle (up to approximately 18 months of age) during their first grazing season—in July–October in temperate and January–March in tropical and subtropical regions.

Pre-Type II ostertagiosis—occurs during the time period larvae are arrested; clinical signs are usually absent; seasonally, occurs in late fall in temperate and late spring and summer in tropical and subtropical regions.

Type II ostertagiosis—occurs months after the ingestion of larvae; emergence of larvae is synchronous, cellular destruction is synchronous, and a clinically more severe disease results with higher mortalities; generally seen in animals 2–4 years of age; seasonally, occurs in February–May in temperate and September–December in tropical and subtropical regions.

- Haemonchosis in sheep and goats

  Both L_4 and adults are voracious blood-feeders, which can lead to normocytic, hypochromic anemia.

Hypoalbuminemia associated with blood loss results in accumulation of fluids in abomasal wall and peripheral edema (most often manifested as "bottle jaw").

Abomasitis resulting from infection may interfere with digestibility and absorption of protein, calcium, and phosphorus.

Petechial to ecchymotic hemorrhages may be seen on mucosal surface of abomasum.

Acute disease—clinical signs include anemia, dark feces, submandibular edema, sudden death.

Chronic disease—clinical signs include inappetence, weight loss or decreased weight gain, anemia; death may occur as a result of depleted protein and iron stores.

Diagnosis

ANTEMORTEM

- Clinical signs are very nonspecific and of little help.

- Knowing the grazing history and seasonal occurrence of parasitism in an area may be helpful.

- Can find trichostrongyle-type eggs on fecal flotation (Figures 4–1 and 4–5).

- Eggs are oval, thin-shelled, grayish in color, $70–110 \times 30–50$ µm, containing morula with 16–32 cells; eggs of *Ostertagia*, *Teladorsagia*, *Haemonchus*, and *Trichostrongylus* (as well as *Cooperia*, *Oesophagostomum*,

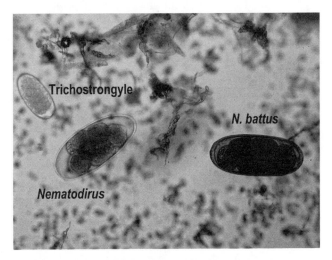

Figure 4–5   Fecal flotation from a sheep with two types of nematodirid eggs and a trichostrongyle-type egg (100×).

and *Chabertia*) are very similar and difficult to differentiate; therefore, must be categorized as trichostrongyle-type and not specific genus or species.

- Definitive diagnosis can be made on identification of infective larvae recovered from coproculture (usually not performed by the practitioner).

POSTMORTEM

- Because of their size, most of these nematodes are missed on gross necropsy.

- *Haemonchus* is the largest nematode in this group (up to 3.0 cm in length), *Ostertagia* and *Teladorsagia* are mid-sized (up to 1.2 cm in length), and *Trichostrongylus* is the smallest (up to 0.8 cm in length).

- Adult *Haemonchus* have a white reproductive tract that spirals around the red (blood-filled) intestine giving a barberpole appearance (hence the common name "barberpole worm").

- The "moroccan leather" appearance of the abomasum is pathognomonic for *Ostertagia* in cattle; petechial or ecchymotic hemorrhages in the abomasum may indicate *Haemonchus* in cattle, sheep, and goats.

Treatment and Control

- See Table 4–3 for anthelmintics; anthelmintic resistance in sheep is an enormous problem in many areas of the world; anthelmintic resistance in cattle occurs, but is not yet as widespread.

Table 4–3 Partial List of Anthelmintics for Cattle and Sheep

Active Ingredient	Dosage (mg/kg)	Route	Trichostrongyles	Arrested larvae	Nematodirus	Oesophagostomum	Bunostomum	Strongyloides	Trichuris	Dictyocaulus	Thelazia	Moniezia	Fasciola
Cattle													
Morantel	See label	In feed	✓		✓	✓							
Albendazole	10	Oral	✓	✓	✓	✓	✓			✓		✓	✓
Oxfendazole	4.5	Oral	✓	✓	✓	✓	✓			✓		✓[1]	
Fenbendazole	5	Oral	✓	✓[1]	✓	✓	✓			✓			
Ivermectin[2]	0.2	SQ	✓	✓	✓	✓	✓			✓			
Doramectin[3]	0.2	SQ	✓	✓	✓	✓	✓	✓		✓			
Eprinomectin	0.5	Pour-on	✓	✓	✓	✓	✓	✓	✓	✓	✓		

Moxidectin	0.5	Pour-on	✓	✓	✓	✓		✓	
Clorsulon	7	Oral							✓
Sheep									
Levamisole	See label	Oral	✓	✓	✓			✓	
Ivermectin	0.2	Oral	✓	✓	✓	✓	✓	✓	

1 Dosage of 10 mg/kg needed.

2 Pour-on and sustained release bolus formulations also available; spectrum of activity and dosage depend on formulation.

3 Pour-on formulation also available; spectrum of activity and dosage different than injectable formulation.

- Control programs must be tailored to the individual situation; control should not rely solely on anthelmintics; judicious use of drugs at key times of the year combined with improved pasture management are essential ingredients of integrated parasite control programs; an understanding of the epidemiology of the parasites in question is key to a successful program.

Small Intestine

COOPERIA SPP.

- Worldwide distribution in grazing ruminants; low significance alone; contributes to enteritis of mixed trichostrongylid infections.

Life Cycle

- Direct.
- Life cycle essentially the same as for *Haemonchus, Ostertagia,* and *Trichostrongylus.*

Pathogenesis and Clinical Signs

- Contributes to catarrhal enteritis; clinical signs may include diarrhea, rough hair coat, decreased weight gain, inappetence.

Diagnosis

ANTEMORTEM

- Generally not diagnosing *Cooperia* alone, but, mixed trichostrongyle infections.

- Knowing the grazing history and seasonal occurrence of parasitism in an area may be helpful.

- Can find trichostrongyle-type eggs on fecal flotation (see Figures 4–1 and 4–5).

- Eggs are oval, thin-shelled, grayish in color, 68–82 × 34–42 µm, containing morula with 16–32 cells; eggs of *Ostertagia, Teladorsagia, Haemonchus,* and *Trichostrongylus* (as well as *Cooperia, Oesophagostomum,* and *Chabertia*) are very similar and difficult to differentiate; therefore, must be categorized as trichostrongyle-type and not specific genus or species.

- Definitive diagnosis can be made on identification of infective larvae recovered from coproculture (usually not performed by the practitioner).

POSTMORTEM
- Because of their size, most of these nematodes are missed on gross necropsy.

- *Cooperia* is up to 0.8 cm in length; found in proximal small intestine.

Treatment and Control

- See Table 4–3 for anthelmintics.

- Concepts regarding control are as for abomasal nematodes.

NEMATODIRUS SPP.
- Includes *Nematodirus battus, N. filicollis, N. spathiger* in sheep, and *N. helvetianus* in cattle.

- Distribution tends towards temperate regions in domestic and sylvatic ruminants; may be locally common; variable significance (species dependent).

Life Cycle

- Direct.
- Eggs are passed in the feces; L_1 develops to infective L_3 within the egg; development and hatching of L_3 may (*N. battus*) or may not (*N. spathiger, N. filicollis*) be seasonally constrained by temperature.
- Ruminants acquire infection by ingestion of L_3; extra-intestinal migration does not occur; develops to adults in small intestine.
- Prepatent period is 2–4 weeks.
- Eggs and hatched L_3 resistant to adverse environmental conditions; can survive overwinter; *N. battus* eggs must overwinter before they can hatch.
- In Britain, temperature influences on the hatching of eggs of *N. battus* concentrates larvae during the spring, with a second wave in the fall; lambs are exposed to a large number of larvae in a short period of time in spring; mass hatching of larvae has not been shown to occur in North America.

Pathogenesis and Clinical Signs

- Except for *N. battus*, generally not considered pathogenic; heavy infections of *N. helvetianus* in dairy calves may cause generalized unthriftiness.

- Catarrhal enteritis is associated with *N. battus* infections; clinical signs include a sudden loss of thrift followed by a severe diarrhea; death can result within 2 days after the onset of clinical signs; losses may continue for several weeks.

Diagnosis

ANTEMORTEM

- Generic diagnosis can be made by finding eggs on fecal flotation (Figure 4–5).
- Eggs are ovoid to football shaped, 150–230 × 80–100 μm, containing morula with 4–8 dark, round cells; may be yellowish-brown in color (*N. battus*).

POSTMORTEM

- Worms are mid- to large-sized (up to 2.5 cm in length); found in proximal small intestine.

Treatment and Control

- See Table 4–3 for anthelmintics; concepts regarding control are as for abomasal nematodes.

STRONGYLOIDES PAPILLOSUS

- Worldwide distribution, especially in tropical regions; low significance; may cause cutaneous larval migrans in humans.
- Common name: threadworm.

Life Cycle

- Direct.
- Life cycle as for *S. ransomi*; primary route of infection for cattle appears to be transmammary; primary route for sheep is percutaneous.

Pathogenesis and Clinical Signs

- Infection in older animals inapparent and usually so in young animals as well; disease, when it does occur, is present only in young animals.
- Infections can cause erosion of the intestinal mucosa; clinical signs may include anorexia, decreased weight gain or weight loss, diarrhea; larvae may be associated with the introduction of bacteria through the inter-digital skin, leading to foot rot.

Diagnosis

ANTEMORTEM

- Eggs may be found on fecal flotation; even though *S. papillosus* eggs are smaller, must use fresh feces to avoid confusion with larvated trichostrongyle-type eggs.
- Eggs are thin-shelled, oval, 40–60 × 20–35 μm, each containing a fully developed larva.

POSTMORTEM

- Adult worms are embedded in the mucosa of the small intestine; worms are extremely small in size (up to 6 mm in length) and will be missed at necropsy unless mucosal scrapings are examined under a microscope.

Treatment and Control

- See Table 4–3 for anthelmintics.
- Maintain clean, dry stalls if animals are housed.

BUNOSTOMUM PHLEBOTOMUM

- Worldwide distribution in cattle; sporadic occurrence but highly pathogenic.
- Common name: hookworm.

Life Cycle

- Direct.
- Eggs passed in feces; L_1 develops and hatches; infective L_3 develops in approximately 7 days.
- Transmission occurs primarily through percutaneous route with pulmonary-tracheal migration as for *Ancylostoma* (see Dog and Cat section); peroral route may also occur in which case extra-intestinal migration also occurs.
- Prepatent period is 60–72 days; may live 1–2 years.

Pathogenesis and Clinical Signs

- Migrating larvae cause dermatitis and pruritis; may result in intense scratching.

- Feeding activities cause severe blood loss and hypoproteinemia; clinical signs include anemia, weight loss or decreased weight gain, emaciation, diarrhea with mucus and blood, and submandibular edema ("bottle jaw"); may result in death.

- Infections generally more severe in calves (5–8 months old); adults may harbor infections with no apparent clinical signs.

Diagnosis

ANTEMORTEM

- Eggs may be found on fecal flotation.

- Eggs are oval, 79–117 × 47–70 µm, containing morula with 4–8 cells.

POSTMORTEM

- Adult worms are grayish white, stout, up to 2.8 cm in length; anterior end is bent dorsally resulting in "hook"; found in proximal portion of the small intestine.

Treatment and Control

- See Table 4–3 for anthelmintics; concepts regarding control are as for abomasal nematodes.

AONCHOTHECA BOVIS

- Worldwide distribution in domestic ruminants; low significance.

Life Cycle

- Direct.
- Eggs are passed in feces, develop to infective stage, and are ingested by the definitive host; mature in small intestine.
- Prepatent period is unknown.

Pathogenesis and Clinical Signs

- No pathological problems are associated with this parasite; primary importance is the ability to distinguish eggs of this parasite from those of *Trichuris*.

Diagnosis

ANTEMORTEM
- Eggs may be found on fecal flotation.
- Eggs are typical capillarid-type (Figure 4–6), barrel-shaped with reduced polar plugs, colorless to yellow, $45–50 \times 22–25$ μm; may be slightly asymmetrical in shape.

POSTMORTEM
- Adults are found in the small intestine; however, because they are quite thin, generally are not seen on gross necropsy.

Treatment and Control

- Generally do not treat cattle for this parasite.

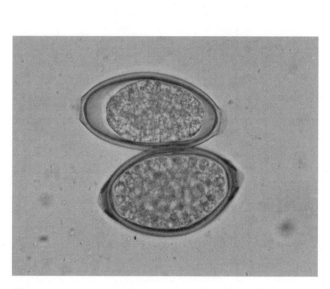

Figure 4–6 Fecal flotation showing a typical appearance of capillarid-type eggs (600×).

Cecum and Large Intestine

OESOPHAGOSTOMUM SPP.

- Includes *Oesophagostomum radiatum* (cattle), *O. venulosum* (cattle, sheep, goats), *O. columbianum* (sheep, goats).
- Worldwide distribution in cattle, sheep, goats, and other domestic and sylvatic ruminants; moderate significance, especially in tropical and subtropical regions.
- Common name: nodular worm.

Life Cycle

- Direct.
- Life cycle essentially as described for nodular worm of pigs.
- Prepatent period is 28–41 days, depending on species present.

Pathogenesis and Clinical Signs

- In all ruminants, developing larvae may cause severe inflammatory reactions resulting in nodular formation; nodules are usually 1–5 mm in diameter and are evident on both the serosal and mucosal side of the gut wall; nodules will caseate and calcify with time; nodule formation may not be associated with *O. venulosum* infections.
- Cattle

    Inflammation and nodular formation can cause loss of cellular tight junctions leading to leakage of blood and plasma proteins.

Clinical signs may include edema, anemia, profuse watery diarrhea, weight loss, or decreased weight gain; death may result.

Repeated infections may elicit a type III hypersensitivity reaction in the gut wall.

- Sheep

  Nodules do not occur unless prior exposure and sensitization have occurred.

  Nodules can cause acute ulcerative colitis and may interfere with digestion, absorption, and peristalsis.

  Clinical signs may include inappetence, emaciation, anemia, and mucoid to bloody diarrhea; death may result.

Diagnosis

ANTEMORTEM

- Eggs may be found on fecal flotation.
- Eggs are thin-shelled, oval, 88–105 × 44–65 μm, contain morula with 16–32 cells; may be difficult to differentiate from trichostrongyle-type eggs.
- Definitive diagnosis through identification of infective larvae recovered from coproculture (usually not performed by the practitioner).

POSTMORTEM

- Adult worms are white, stout, up to 2.2 cm in length; found in cecum and colon.

Treatment and Control

- See Table 4–3 for anthelmintics.
- Concepts regarding control are as for abomasal nematodes.

CHABERTIA OVINA

- Worldwide distribution in sheep, goats, and other ruminants; may be locally significant.
- Common name: large-mouthed bowel worm.

Life Cycle

- Direct.
- Eggs passed in feces; L_1 hatches; develops to infective L_3 within 5 days, depending on environmental conditions.
- Ruminants acquire infection by ingestion of infective L_3; L_3 migrate into the wall of the small intestine; develop and molt to L_4 within the wall, then return to lumen and migrate to cecum; molt to immature adult and pass to the colon where they mature.
- Prepatent period is approximately 7 weeks.

Pathogenesis and Clinical Signs

- L_4 and adults attach to colonic mucosa; feed on plugs of tissue that leads to colitis.

- Clinical signs may be inapparent; when present, may include a bloody, mucoid diarrhea, anemia, decreased wool production, death.

Diagnosis

ANTEMORTEM

- Eggs may be found on fecal flotation.
- Eggs are thin-shelled, oval, 90–105 × 50–55 μm, contain morula with 16–32 cells; may be difficult to differentiate from trichostrongyle-type eggs.
- Definitive diagnosis through identification of infective larvae recovered from coproculture (usually not performed by the practitioner).

POSTMORTEM

- Adult worms are white, stout, up to 2 cm in length, anterior end bent slightly ventral; found firmly attached to mucosal surface of colon.
- Can be differentiated from *Oesophagostomum* spp. by the presence of a large buccal capsule.

Treatment and Control

- Ivermectin at 0.2 mg per kg is approved for sheep.
- Concepts regarding control are as for abomasal nematodes.

TRICHURIS SPP.

- Numerous species described; those important in North America include *Trichuris ovis*, *T. skrjabini*, and *T. discolor*.
- Worldwide distribution; low to moderate significance.

Life Cycle

- Direct.
- Life cycle essentially as described for *T. suis*.
- Prepatent period 7–9 weeks for *T. ovis*; unknown for others.

Pathogenesis and Clinical Signs

- Infections are usually asymptomatic; if clinical signs do occur, may include inappetence and bloody diarrhea.

Diagnosis

ANTEMORTEM

- Typical trichurid-type eggs may be found on fecal flotation (see Figure 4–3).
- Eggs are 60–80 × 25–42 μm.

POSTMORTEM

- Adult worms are whip-like in appearance, 5–8 cm in length; found attached to mucosal surface of cecum and colon.

Treatment and Control

- See Table 4–3 for anthelmintics.
- Control of trichostrongylid nematodes generally also controls trichurids.

Dogs and Cats

Esophagus and Stomach

SPIROCERCA LUPI

- Worldwide distribution primarily in tropical and sub-tropical areas; in domestic and wild canids and wild felids although rare in domestic cats; sporadic occurrence; moderate significance.

Life Cycle

- Indirect.
- Intermediate hosts: coprophagous beetles.
- Paratenic hosts: a variety of mammals, birds, lizards, toads.
- Larvated eggs are passed in feces and ingested by the intermediate host; L_1 hatches and develops to infective L_3.
- Definitive host becomes infected by ingesting intermediate or paratenic host containing infective L_3; larvae penetrate the gastric wall and migrate in the walls of the gastroepiploic and gastric arteries to the

celiac artery to the aorta; molt to immature adults, then migrate through the connective tissue to the wall of the adjacent esophagus.

- Prepatent period is 4–6 months.

Pathogenesis and Clinical Signs

- Infections may be inapparent.
- Migration in the aorta produces hemorrhage, inflammation, fibrotic nodules, necrosis of the vessel wall, and scarring; stenosis or aneurysms may result.
- Adults cause large granulomatous nodules that develop cavities containing milky fluid and worms in fibrous tissue; nodules may interfere with swallowing or compress adjacent trachea; chronic inflammation may cause esophageal neuromuscular degeneration; esophageal fibrosarcomas, osteosarcomas, and hypertrophic pulmonary osteopathy have been associated with chronic infections.
- Clinical signs may include vomiting, dysphagia, hemoptysis, sudden death.

Diagnosis

ANTEMORTEM
- Eggs may be found on fecal flotation using 33% zinc sulfate or sugar solution with a specific gravity of >1.25; may also find eggs on flotation of vomitus.

- Eggs are thick-shelled, 30–37 × 11–15 μm, each containing a larva.

POSTMORTEM

- Worms are bright red, stout, 3–8 cm in length; found entwined in large nodules in the lower esophagus, occasionally stomach.

Treatment and Control

- Diethylcarbamazine at 20 mg per kg daily for 10 days has been effective.
- Prevent predation and scavenging whenever possible.

PHYSALOPTERA SPP.

- Worldwide distribution in felids, canids, and other mammals; sporadic occurrence and moderate significance in domestic cats and dogs.

Life Cycle

- Indirect.
- Intermediate hosts: beetles, cockroaches, crickets.
- Paratenic hosts: snakes; possibly frogs and mice.
- Larvated eggs are passed in feces, ingested by the intermediate host in which they develop to infective L_3.

- Definitive host becomes infected by ingesting intermediate or paratenic host containing infective L_3; larvae do not migrate beyond the gastric mucosa; mature to adult.

- Prepatent period is 41–83 days, depending on species.

Pathogenesis and Clinical Signs

- Adults are firmly attached to and feed on the mucosa of stomach; may also suck blood; causes ulcerations, hemorrhage, and catarrhal gastritis.

- Clinical signs may include vomiting and anorexia; less common are dark, tarry feces.

Diagnosis

ANTEMORTEM

- Eggs may be found on fecal flotation; must use solution of >1.25 specific gravity.

- Eggs are thick-shelled, smooth, 49–59 × 30–34 μm, each containing a fully developed larva.

- May find adults in vomitus; must differentiate from ascarids; can do this by breaking open female worm and examining eggs.

- Can see worms in stomach on endoscopy.

POSTMORTEM

- Stout worms, up to 4.8 cm in length; found attached to gastric mucosa.

Treatment and Control

- Fenbendazole at 50 mg per kg daily for 3 days has been successful in dogs; ivermectin at 0.2 mg per kg once or two doses of pyrantel pamoate at 5 mg per kg at 3-week intervals have been used in cats.

AONCHOTHECA PUTORII

- Primarily European and North American distribution in mustelids, bobcats, raccoons; occasionally reported in cats in the United States; low significance.

Life Cycle

- Details unknown; presumed to be similar to *A. bovis*; earthworms may ingest eggs.

Pathogenesis and Clinical Signs

- May be associated with gastritis.

Diagnosis

ANTEMORTEM

- Eggs may be found on fecal flotation.
- Eggs are capillarid-type (see Figure 4–6) with flattened sides and reduced polar plugs, colorless to yellow, 56–72 × 23–32 μm; surface has net-like appearance; may be slightly asymmetrical in shape.

POSTMORTEM

- Adults are found in the stomach and small intestine; however, because they are quite small, generally are not seen on gross necropsy.

Treatment and Control

- Ivermectin at 0.3 mg per kg orally appears to be effective.

Small Intestine

ANCYLOSTOMA SPP.

- Includes *A. caninum* (dogs), *A. tubaeforme* (cats), and *A. braziliense* (dogs and cats).

- Worldwide distribution; highly significant to both veterinary medicine and public health.

- Common name: hookworm

Life Cycle

- Direct; indirect with paratenic host.

- Eggs passed in feces; L_1 develops and hatches; infective L_3 develops in as few as 5–8 days; conditions conducive to larval development include well-drained soils, shaded areas, warmth, and humidity.

- Routes of transmission include (Table 4–4):

    Percutaneous—In general, the most common route of transmission; larvae penetrate skin and enter circulatory system passing through the

Table 4–4   Transmission Routes for the Common Hookworms of Dogs and Cats

Parasite	Routes of Transmission			
	Percuta-neous	Peroral	Paratenic Host	Trans-mammary
A. caninum	Yes	Yes	Yes	Major route for pups
A. tubae-forme	Yes	Yes	Yes	No
A. bra-ziliense	Yes	Yes	Yes	No
U. steno-cephala	Uncom-mon	Yes	Yes	No

heart to the lungs; penetrate alveoli, are coughed up and swallowed, mature in lumen of small intestine (pulmonary-tracheal route).

Peroral—Ingested larvae enter glands of the stomach and crypts of the small intestine, molt to L_4, return to the lumen of the small intestine, and mature.

Ingestion of paratenic hosts—A form of peroral transmission.

Transmammary—Another form of peroral transmission that occurs with *A. caninum* (not *A. tubaeforme* or *A. braziliense*); following exposure of currently infected or immunologically competent older dogs, larvae may inhibit development during migration in skeletal muscles or gut wall;

in female dogs, larvae are "reactivated" during the last 2 weeks of pregnancy, migrate to the mammary gland, and are ingested by nursing pups; larvae then mature in the pups as for the peroral route; "reactivated" larvae may also enter the dam's small intestine and mature; most common route of transmission for puppies.

- Prepatent period is 2–4 weeks, depending on the route of transmission.

Pathogenesis and Clinical Signs

- Dermatitis and pneumonia associated with migrating larvae may occur, but are uncommon.

- The most common disease problem is a hypochromic, normocytic anemia which is a result of the feeding activities of the parasite; as iron reserves are depleted, hypochromic, microcytic anemia ensues; mucous membranes are pale; feces may be soft to liquid and quite dark as a result of the partially digested blood.

- Severity of disease associated with infection depends on the number and species of parasites, and age and immune status of host; *A. caninum* more pathogenic than the other two species.

- Clinical disease in dogs associated with *A. caninum* may take one of four forms:

  1. *Peracute*—Results from transmammary transmission; occurs in very young pups that are healthy at first then suddenly deteriorate.

2. *Acute*—Results from sudden exposure of susceptible older pups or adults to overwhelming numbers of larvae; severe anemia occurs.

3. *Chronic (compensated)*—Occurs in immunocompetent animals not exposed to overwhelming numbers of larvae; clinical signs usually are not apparent.

4. *Secondary (decompensated)*—Occurs in older animals secondary to other problems; severe anemia results.

- Clinical disease associated with *A. tubaeforme* in cats is not common.

- *Ancylostoma braziliense* causes less blood loss than *A. caninum* and is considered to be much less pathogenic.

- Cutaneous larval migrans (CLM; also called "creeping eruption") in humans is most often associated with *A. braziliense*; the disease is characterized by serpentine, erythematous tracks and pruritis, a result of the immunological response to the migrating larvae in the skin.

- Occasionally, *A. caninum* may mature to adults in small intestine of humans.

Diagnosis

ANTEMORTEM
- Eggs may be found on fecal flotation.
- Eggs are thin-shelled, oval, 55–90 × 34–45 μm, containing morula with 2–8 cells (Figure 4–7).

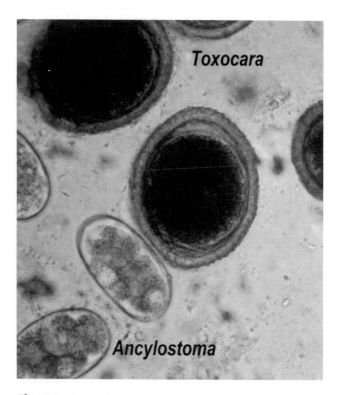

Figure 4–7 Fecal flotation from a dog with both *A. caninum* and *T. canis* (400×).

- In the case of peracute hookworm disease, eggs will *not* be found on fecal flotation because the profound anemia occurs before adults begin laying eggs.

POSTMORTEM
- Adult worms are red, up to 2.8 cm in length; anterior end is bent dorsally resulting in "hook"; found in small intestine, especially the jejunum.
- Genera can be differentiated based on number of teeth in the buccal cavity.

Treatment and Control
- See Tables 4–5 and 4–6 for anthelmintics; supportive therapy is often the more immediate concern but do not delay anthelmintic treatment.
- Dogs: to prevent transmammary transmission, infected bitches can be treated with fenbendazole at 50 mg per kg daily from day 40 of pregnancy through day 14 of lactation or ivermectin at 0.5 mg per kg given 4–9 days prior to whelping followed by a second treatment 10 days later; use concrete-floored kennels; remove feces at least 2 times per week; keep floors clean and dry; deworming schedule for pups is as for ascarids; be sure to use an anthelmintic effective against migrating larvae; prevent predation and scavenging whenever possible.
- Cats: avoid overcrowding; prevent predation and scavenging whenever possible; deworming schedule for kittens is as for ascarids.

Table 4–5 Partial List of Anthelmintics for Dogs

Active Ingredient	Dosage (mg/kg)	Route	Ascarids	Ancylostoma	Uncaria	Trichuris	Taenia	Dipylidium	Echinococcus
Piperazine[1]	See label	Oral	✓						
Pyrantel pamoate	5	Oral	✓	✓	✓				
Fenbendazole	50[2]	Oral	✓	✓	✓	✓	✓		
Febantel[3]	10	Oral	✓	✓	✓	✓			
Epsiprantel	2.5	Oral					✓	✓	
Praziquantel	See label	Oral, IM					✓	✓	✓

[1] Repeat in 30 days or as necessary.
[2] Administered daily for 3 days.
[3] Product is in combination with praziquantel or praziquantel and pyrantel pamoate.

Table 4–6 Partial List of Anthelmintics for Cats

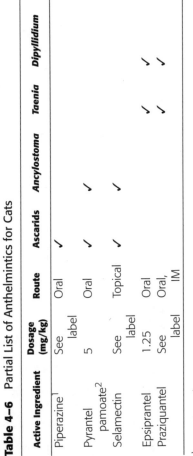

Active Ingredient	Dosage (mg/kg)	Route	Ascarids	Ancylostoma	Taenia	Dipyllidium
Piperazine[1]	See label	Oral	✓			
Pyrantel pamoate[2]	5	Oral	✓	✓		
Selamectin	See label	Topical	✓	✓		
Epsiprantel	1.25	Oral			✓	✓
Praziquantel	See label	Oral, IM			✓	✓

[1] Repeat in 30 days or as necessary.
[2] Product is in combination with praziquantel.

- Prevention of cutaneous larval migrans: recommendations include prevent infections in dogs and cats, keep pets from defecating in public places, reduce the number of strays, and educate the public about the disease.

UNCINARIA STENOCEPHALA (NORTHERN HOOKWORM OF DOGS AND CATS)

- Found in northern temperate areas; moderate to low significance.

Life Cycle

- Direct; indirect with paratenic host.
- Eggs passed in feces; L_1 develops and hatches; infective L_3 develops in approximately 1 week.
- Transmission occurs through the peroral route; no extra-intestinal migration; percutaneous infection is uncommon; transmammary infection does not occur (see Table 4–4).
- Prepatent period is approximately 2 weeks.

Pathogenesis and Clinical Signs

- Generally not associated with severe blood loss; may be some catarrhal inflammation; clinical signs may not be apparent.

Diagnosis

ANTEMORTEM
- Eggs may be found on fecal flotation.
- Eggs are thin-shelled, oval, 65–80 × 45–50 µm, containing morula with 8 cells.

POSTMORTEM
- Adult worms are white, up to 1.2 cm in length; anterior end is bent dorsally resulting in "hook"; found in posterior one-third of the small intestine.
- Can be differentiated from species of *Ancylostoma* based on the presence of cutting plates rather than teeth in buccal cavity.

Treatment and Control

- See Table 4–5 for anthelmintics.

TOXASCARIS LEONINA
- Worldwide distribution in dogs, cats; commonly diagnosed, but of moderate significance.

Life Cycle

- Direct; indirect with paratenic host.
- Eggs passed in feces; infective L_3 develops within the egg in approximately 1 week.
- Transmission occurs through ingestion of eggs containing infective L_3 or ingestion of paratenic rodent

host (may be the most important route; Table 4–7); extra-intestinal migration does not occur; larvae penetrate the mucosa of the small intestine, molt to L_4, then return to the lumen and mature to adults.

- Prepatent period is 7–11 weeks if eggs are ingested; prepatent period is shortened by approximately 2 weeks if infection results from eating paratenic host.

Pathogenesis and Clinical Signs

- Clinical signs include unthriftiness, pot-bellied appearance, intermittent diarrhea.

Diagnosis

ANTEMORTEM

- Eggs may be found on fecal flotation.
- Eggs are subspherical, light, colorless, with a smooth outer shell, 75–85 × 60–75 µm in size, single cell present, which does not fill the egg (Figure 4–8).

POSTMORTEM

- Adult worms are large, white, up to 10 cm in length; found in small intestine.
- Can be differentiated from *Toxocara* spp. based on cervical alae, esophagus, and male tail.

Treatment and Control

- See Tables 4–5 and 4–6 for anthelmintics.

Table 4–7 Transmission Routes for the Common Ascarids of Dogs and Cats

| Parasite | Routes of Transmission | | | |
	Peroral	Paratenic Host	Transmammary	Prenatal
T. canis	Yes	Yes	Minor route	Major route for pups
T. mystax	Yes	Yes	Major route for kittens	No
T. leonina	Yes	Major route	No	No

- See *Toxocara* for deworming schedule of pups and kittens; prevent predation and scavenging whenever possible.

TOXOCARA SPP.

- Includes *T. canis* (canine ascarid) and *T. mystax* (feline ascarid).
- Worldwide distribution in dogs and cats; commonly diagnosed; moderate significance to veterinary medicine but highly significant to public health.

Life Cycle

- Direct; indirect with paratenic host.

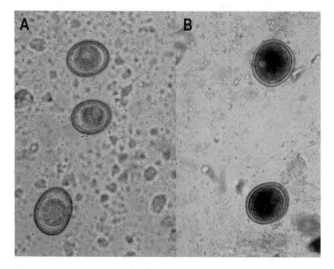

Figure 4–8   Eggs of *T. leonina* (A) and *T. canis* (B) (100×).

- Eggs passed in feces; infective L_3 develops within the egg in 3–4 weeks.
- Routes of transmission include (see Table 4–7):

  Peroral—Ingestion of infective L_3 in eggs; for *T. canis* in young pups (1 month old or younger), larvae hatch within the gut and undergo hepatic-pulmonary migration as for *A. suum*; prepatent period is approximately 28 days; for *T. canis* in older pups, larvae hatch, migrate to the lungs, but continue to the somatic tissues where they inhibit development; for *T. mystax* in cats, tendency for arrested development does not increase with age; prepatent period is 2 months.

  Prenatal—Larvae are "reactivated" from tissues of dam, migrate to the lungs of pups in utero during the last trimester, molt to L_4, mature in small intestine after birth; prepatent period is 3–5 weeks; the most important mode of transmission of *T. canis* of dogs; does not occur in *T. mystax* of cats; "reactivated" larvae may also migrate to the small intestine of bitch and mature.

  Transmammary—A form of peroral transmission; "reactivated" larvae migrate to mammary glands and are ingested by the nursing pups or kittens; minor significance in transmission of *T. canis*; most important mode of transmission of *T. mystax*; transmammary transmission results in development and maturation as for *T. leonina* (i.e., no extra-intestinal migration); prepatent period is approximately 21 days.

Ingestion of paratenic host—Another form of per-oral transmission occurring for both *T. canis* and *T. mystax*; numerous animals can be paratenic hosts; this mode of transmission results in development and maturation as for *T. leonina* (i.e., no extra-intestinal migration); prepatent period is approximately 21 days.

Pathogenesis and Clinical Signs

- Verminous pneumonia, associated with larval *T. canis*, may occur in pups.

- Adults of both species may cause mechanical damage to the small intestine; in older animals, infections are often inapparent.

- Clinical signs, especially in pups and kittens, may include vomiting, diarrhea, general unthriftiness; intestinal obstruction can occur, but is not common; death may result from severe prenatal or lactogenic infections in pups and kittens within 2–3 weeks of birth.

- Larvae can cause visceral larval migrans (VLM) or ocular larval migrans (OLM) in humans; embryonated eggs are ingested, hatch, and larvae continuously migrate through various tissues until trapped by inflammatory reaction; granuloma formation results with larval death; character and severity of problems caused depend on the tissues the larvae are in, the number of migrating larvae, and the frequency of reinfection.

Diagnosis

ANTEMORTEM

- Eggs may be found on fecal flotation.

- Eggs are subspherical, yellow-brown outer shell that is roughly pitted, 75–90 μm (*T. canis*) or 65–75 μm (*T. mystax*), containing dark, single cell that fills interior of egg (see Figures 4–7 and 4–8).

POSTMORTEM

- Adult worms are large, white, 3–10 cm (*T. mystax*) or 10–18 cm (*T. canis*) in length; found in small intestine.

Treatment and Control

- See Tables 4–5 and 4–6 for anthelmintics.

- Dogs: for control of both hookworms and ascarids, initiate treatment in pups at 2 weeks of age; repeat at 4, 6, and 8 weeks of age; treat bitch concurrently.

- Cats: for control of both hookworms and ascarids, initiate treatment in kittens at 3 weeks of age; repeat at 8 and 10 weeks of age; treat queen concurrently.

- Recommendations for prevention of human exposure are the same as for cutaneous larval migrans.

BAYLISASCARIS PROCYONIS

- Distributed throughout most of the continental United States in raccoons; introduced to Europe with raccoons; highly significant to veterinary medicine and public health.

Life Cycle

- Direct; indirect with paratenic host.

- Eggs passed in feces; infective L_3 develops within the egg in approximately 1 week.

- Transmission occurs through ingestion of eggs containing infective L_3 or ingestion of paratenic host; extra-intestinal migration does not occur; larvae penetrate the mucosa of the small intestine, molt to L_4, return to the lumen, and mature to adults.

- Prepatent period is 50–76 days if eggs ingested, 32–38 days if paratenic host is ingested.

- Raccoons tend to defecate in certain areas called latrines; thus, egg numbers can be high in discrete areas.

Pathogenesis and Clinical Signs

- Clinical signs in definitive host are uncommon.

- Primary significance is in paratenic hosts in which a severe, fatal neurologic disorder occurs; a wide variety of paratenic hosts, including gray squirrels, ground squirrels, rabbits, various birds, dogs, and humans, may be infected.

- Occasionally, in dogs, may develop to maturity and pass eggs; dogs tend to defecate anywhere and eggs can therefore be dispersed to more areas, increasing chance contact with humans.

Diagnosis

ANTEMORTEM
- Eggs may be found on fecal flotation (raccoon, dog).
- Eggs are ovoid, brown, with a finely pitted outer shell, 62–70 × 52–57 μm in size, containing single cell that does not fill the egg.

POSTMORTEM
- Adult worms are large, white, up to 18 cm in length; found in small intestine (raccoon, possibly dog).
- In other hosts, identifying characteristic features of larvae in histological sections or those recovered from digests of brain or other tissues.

Treatment and Control

- Anthelmintics effective against *Toxocara canis* appear to be effective against *B. procyonis* in raccoons; piperazine at 220 mg per kg is effective against infections in dogs; treatment of larval disease is difficult and generally unrewarding.

STRONGYLOIDES STERCORALIS, S. TUMEFACIENS
- Worldwide distribution, especially in tropical regions; moderate significance; *S. stercoralis* may contribute to cutaneous larval migrans in humans.

- Common name: threadworm.

Life Cycle

- Direct.
- Life cycle as described for *S. ransomi* except L_1 hatch from egg in intestinal tract and are passed with the feces.
- Routes of infection include only percutaneous and autoinfection; autoinfection occurs when L_1 in intestine develops to infective L_3 before passing out of host; penetrates mucosa of rectum or perianal skin and migrates as for percutaneous infections.

Pathogenesis and Clinical Signs

- Infection in older animals inapparent and usually so in young animals as well; disease, when it does occur, is present only in young animals.
- Dogs: percutaneous route is most common; dermatitis may occur in response to larvae; catarrhal enteritis with necrosis and sloughing of intestinal mucosa may occur; clinical signs may include moderate to severe mucoid or bloody diarrhea, dehydration, death; generally a kennel problem occurring in summer when weather is hot and humid; larvae of *S. stercoralis* can penetrate human skin, causing cutaneous larval migrans (see description under *Ancylostoma*).

- Cats: percutaneous route most common; for *S. stercoralis*, clinical course of disease as for dog; for *S. tumefaciens*, infections may cause nodular formation on mucosal surface of the colon; clinical signs include diarrhea.

Diagnosis

ANTEMORTEM

- Eggs of *S. tumefaciens* may be found on fecal flotation; must use fresh feces to avoid confusion with larvated hookworm eggs.
- Eggs are thin-shelled, oval, 114–124 × 62–68 μm, each containing a fully developed larva.
- For *S. stercoralis*, use Baermann technique to detect L_1 in feces.

POSTMORTEM

- Adult worms are embedded in the mucosa of the small intestine (*S. stercoralis*) or the large intestine (*S. tumefaciens*); worms are extremely small in size (*S. stercoralis* up to 2.2 mm in length) and will be missed at necropsy unless mucosal scrapings are examined under a microscope.

Treatment and Control

- Ivermectin at 0.2 mg per kg, SQ, appears to be useful, but may need to be repeated; thiabendazole at 100–150 mg per kg daily for 3 days repeated weekly until fecals are negative for larvae can also be used in dogs; thiabendazole at 125 mg per kg daily for 3 days has been recommended in cats.

- To avoid human infections with *S. stercoralis*, isolate infected animals; infections tend to recur in dogs so monitor fecals monthly for at least 6 months after the first negative fecal to ensure larval output has ceased.

Large Intestine

TRICHURIS SPP.

- Includes *T. vulpis* in canids, and *T. campanula* and *T. serrata* in cats.
- Worldwide distribution in canids with low to moderate significance; distribution in cats unknown although virtually absent from North America.
- Although rare, *T. vulpis* has been reported in humans.
- Common name: whipworm.

Life Cycle

- Direct.
- Essentially as described for *T. suis*.
- Prepatent period for *T. vulpis* is 11–12 weeks; may live several years.
- Prepatent period for *T. campanula* is 8–13 weeks.

Pathogenesis and Clinical Signs

- Infections with whipworms in cats are rare and apparently nonpathogenic.

- In dogs, typhilitis and colitis may occur in heavy infections; clinical signs may include chronic, mucoid diarrhea with frank blood, colic, inappetance, weight loss, unthriftiness.

Diagnosis

ANTEMORTEM

- Typical trichurid-type eggs may be found on fecal flotation (see Figures 4–3 and 7–1).
- *Trichuris vulpis*: eggs are 70–80 × 30–40 μm.
- *Trichuris campanula*: eggs are 63–85 × 34–39 μm.

POSTMORTEM

- Adults worms are whip-like in appearance, 4.5–7.5 cm (*T. vulpis*) or 2.2–3.1 cm (*T. campanula*) in length; found attached to mucosal surface of cecum and colon.

Treatment and Control

- See Table 4–5 for anthelmintics; retreat in 3 weeks and 3 months.
- Keep kennels dry, remove feces daily, and thoroughly clean all areas at least two times per month.

Poultry and Other Birds

Esophagus and Crop

EUCOLEUS SPP

- Several species exist; those important to North America include *Eucoleus annulatus* and *E. contortus*.

Life Cycle

- Direct or indirect.
- *Eucoleus annulatus* is indirect while *E. contortus* can be direct or indirect (with paratenic host).
- Eggs are passed with the feces; L_1 develops, but does not hatch; eggs ingested by earthworm hatch, but larvae do not develop further.
- Bird acquires infection by ingestion of infective eggs or infected earthworm; larvae penetrate the epithelium of the mouth and esophagus or crop and mature.

Pathogenesis and Clinical Signs

- Mild inflammation and thickening of the crop occurs with light infections; heavier infections cause marked thickening of the crop and esophagus, catarrhal inflammation, and sloughing of the mucosa.
- Clinical signs may include unthriftiness, anorexia, emaciation, and death.

Diagnosis

ANTEMORTEM
- May find capillarid-type eggs on fecal flotation; eggs are of similar size and can be confused with other, less pathogenic, capillarids.

POSTMORTEM
- Generally the method of choice for diagnosis; squash preparation of esophageal or crop wall is examined to see the parasites; if walls are too thick, take deep mucosal scrapings and examine microscopically.

Treatment and Control

- Hygromycin is effective against capillarid nematodes.
- Intensive management has decreased the incidence of most poultry parasites except coccidia; reuse of litter may lead to build-up of high levels of contamination.

Small Intestine

BARUSCAPILLARIA OBSIGNATA
- Probably worldwide distribution; sporadic occurrence.

Life Cycle

- Direct.
- Eggs are passed with the feces; L_1 develops, but does not hatch.

- Bird acquires infection by ingestion of infective eggs; larvae penetrate the epithelium of the small intestine.

Pathogenesis and Clinical Signs

- Mild inflammation and thickening of the small intestine occur; heavy infections cause catarrhal inflammation and sloughing of the mucosa.
- Clinical signs may include unthriftiness, anorexia, emaciation, and death.

Diagnosis

ANTEMORTEM
- May find capillarid-type eggs on fecal flotation; eggs are of similar size and can be confused with other, less pathogenic, capillarids.

POSTMORTEM
- Generally the method of choice for diagnosis; take deep mucosal scrapings of the small intestine and examine microscopically.

Treatment and Control

- See comments for *Eucoleus.*

ASCARIDIA SPP.
- Includes *A. galli* in chickens and game birds, *A. columbae* in pigeons, and *A. dissimilis* in turkeys.

- Worldwide distribution; moderate to high significance.

Life Cycle

- Direct; indirect with paratenic host.
- Eggs passed in feces; infective L_3 develops within the egg in 1–2 weeks; larvated eggs may remain viable in the environment for approximately 1 year.
- Transmission occurs through ingestion of eggs containing the infective L_3; extra-intestinal migration does not occur; earthworms may serve as paratenic hosts.
- Prepatent period varies with age of bird; in young birds, prepatent period is approximately 5 and 6 weeks for *A. galli* and *A. columbae*, respectively; in adult birds, prolonged to 8 weeks or longer.
- Infections more prevalent and heavier in young birds; older birds may be carriers.

Pathogenesis and Clinical Signs

- Moderate infections may be inapparent; heavier infections can cause decreased feed intake, catarrhal enteritis, death.
- Clinical signs include off-feed, dull plummage, decreased egg production, diarrhea.

Diagnosis

ANTEMORTEM
- Eggs may be found on fecal flotation.
- Eggs are oval to ellipsoidal, with a thick, smooth shell, 73–92 × 40–60 µm, containing a single cell; similar to *H. gallinarum* in appearance, but somewhat larger.

POSTMORTEM
- Adult worms are white, up to 12 cm in length (varies with species); found in the small intestine.

Treatment and Control

- Piperazine, fenbendazole, and levamisole are effective.
- Prevention is generally through feeding of chicks prophylactic levels of anthelmintics.

Cecae

HETERAKIS GALLINARUM
- Worldwide distribution in galliform and anseriform birds; moderate to high significance.
- Common name: cecal worm.

Life Cycle

- Direct; indirect with paratenic host.
- Eggs passed in feces; infective L_3 develops within the egg in approximately 2 weeks.

- Transmission occurs through ingestion of egg containing infective L_3; eggs hatch in the small intestine and larvae migrate to the cecae where they mature; extra-intesinal migration does not occur; earthworms may serve as paratenic hosts.

- Prepatent period is approximately 4 weeks.

Pathogenesis and Clinical Signs

- Hemorrhages and thickening of the cecal mucosa occur in heavy infections.

- Importance is as a vector for *Histomonas meleagridis*, the causative agent of "blackhead" in turkeys (see Chapter 8).

Diagnosis

ANTEMORTEM
- Eggs may be found on fecal flotation.

- Eggs are ellipsoidal, with a thick, smooth shell, 65–80 µm in size, containing a single cell; similar in appearance to *A. galli* but somewhat smaller.

POSTMORTEM
- Adult worms are white, small, up to 1.5 cm in length; found in cecae.

Treatment and Control

- Same as for *A. galli*.

5

Parasites of the Gastrointestinal Tract II—Acanthocephalans, Cestodes, and Trematodes

Acanthocephalans

Small Intestine

MACRACANTHORHYNCHUS HIRUDINACEUS

- Worldwide distribution in domestic and feral pigs; sporadic occurrence, primarily in pigs in outdoor management situations; occasionally found in dogs, wild carnivores, and humans.

Life Cycle

- Indirect.

- Intermediate host: dung beetles.

- Eggs passed in feces; beetle grubs ingest eggs; acanthor to acanthella to cystacanth in beetle in about 3–6 months.

- Pigs become infected by ingesting infected grub or adult beetle containing cystacanth; parasite attaches to gut wall and matures.

- Prepatent period is 2–3 months; may live 10 or more months.

Pathogenesis and Clinical Signs

- Proboscis embedded in wall of intestine results in inflammation and granuloma formation that is visible from the serosal surface of the intestine; catarrhal enteritis may be present.

- Intestinal perforation resulting in peritonitis rarely occurs.

- Decreased feed intake, diarrhea, decreased weight gain or weight loss, or acute abdominal pain may result.

Diagnosis

ANTEMORTEM

- Eggs in feces; sedimentation techniques preferred as eggs do not float well in most flotation media.

- Eggs are almond shaped, with a thick, dark brown shell that contains the acanthor; approximately 67–110 × 40–65 µm.

POSTMORTEM

- Adults are quite large, 6–40 cm in length, pinkish with transverse wrinkle giving a segmented appearance; proboscis embedded in intestinal wall.

- Superficially resembles *Ascaris suum*; can be differentiated by the presence of a proboscis that is attached to the intestinal wall.

Treatment and Control

- Ivermectin, SQ, at 0.3 mg per kg is effective.

- Prevent access of pigs to intermediate hosts if possible.

Cestodes, Cyclophyllidea
Small Intestine
DIPYLIDIUM CANINUM

- Worldwide distribution in felids and canids, occasionally humans; low significance.

- Common name: double-pored tapeworm.

Life Cycle

- Indirect.

- Intermediate hosts: fleas (*Ctenocephalids felis*, *Pulex irritans*), lice (*Trichodectes canis*).

- Metacestode stage: cysticercoid.

- Prepatent period is 2–3 weeks.

Pathogenesis and Clinical Signs

- Usually nonpathogenic; proglottids may cause pruritis as they migrate in perianal area.

Diagnosis

ANTEMORTEM

- Gravid proglottids, which resemble rice grains when dried, may be found in feces, on pets' hair, or in their bedding; when fresh or rehydrated, shaped like a cucumber seed with a lateral pore on each side (double-pored).

- Eggs, approximately 50 μm in diameter, occur in packets; crush proglottid to demonstrate egg packets; may find packets or individual eggs on fecal flotation (Figure 5–1).

- Individual eggs difficult to differentiate from those of *Taenia* spp.

POSTMORTEM

- Up to 50 cm in length; scolex with four suckers, retractable rostellum armed with three rows of rosethorn-shaped hooks; mature and gravid segments longer than wide, cucumber-seed shaped, double-pored; lives in small intestine.

Treatment and Control

- See Tables 4–5 and 4–6 for treatment.
- Flea and louse control to eliminate the intermediate hosts.

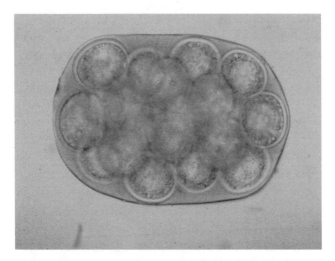

Figure 5–1   Egg packet of *D. caninum* containing at least 17 eggs (400×).

TAENIA SPP.

- Worldwide distribution; moderate to highly significant.
- Over 60 species have been described; only 6–8 regularly seen in veterinary medicine.

Life Cycle

- Indirect.
- See Table 5–1 for intermediate hosts and metacestode type.
- Cysticercus is thin-walled, fluid-filled vesicle containing a single invaginated scolex, range from pea-size (*T. pisiformis*) up to 8 cm (*T. hydatigena*); for every cysticercus ingested by the definitive host, one tapeworm develops.
- Strobilocercus is a variation of the cysticercus; consists of a scolex attached to a long neck attached to the fluid-filled bladder; for every strobilocercus ingested by the definitive host, one tapeworm develops.
- Coenurus is a single, large fluid-filled bladder containing numerous invaginated scolices attached to the inner wall; for every coenurus ingested by the definitive host, several tapeworms can develop.
- Prepatent period is 1–2 months, depending on the species.

Pathogenesis and Clinical Signs

- Infections in the definitive host are generally nonpathogenic.

Table 5–1 Taeniid Tapeworms of Carnivores

Species	Definitive Hosts	Intermediate Hosts	Metacestode Type	Metacestode Site
T. pisiformis	Canids, rare in cats	Lagomorphs	Cysticercus	Abdominal cavity, liver
T. ovis	Canids	Sheep, goats	Cysticercus	Skeletal, cardiac muscles
T. hydatigena	Canids	Domestic and wild ruminants	Cysticercus	Abdominal cavity, liver
T. taeniaeformis	Felids	Rodents	Strobilocercus	Liver
T. multiceps	Canids	Sheep, cattle	Coenurus	Nervous tissue
T. serialis	Canids	Rabbits, rarely cats, humans	Coenurus	Musculature, subcutis
E. granulosus	Canids	Ruminants, macropods, horses, pigs, humans	Hydatid cyst	Primarily liver, lungs
E. multilocularis	Canids, cats	Rodents, horses, pigs, humans	Hydatid cyst	Primarily liver, lungs

- Intermediate hosts:

    Taenia pisiformis: heavy or acute infections may cause digestive disturbances, liver damage, death.

    Taenia ovis: usually nonpathogenic; meat condemnations result in economic loss.

    Taenia hydatigena: may cause liver dysfunction if large numbers are present; liver condemnations result in economic loss.

    Taenia taeniaeformis: usually nonpathogenic; occasionally associated with hepatic sarcomas.

    Taenia multiceps: developing coenurus in CNS causes pressure necrosis; clinical signs may include inappetence, weight loss, head pressing, blindness, circling, and other signs of CNS disorder.

    Taenia serialis: generally nonpathogenic.

Diagnosis

ANTEMORTEM
- Definitive hosts only: gravid proglottids may be found in feces, on pets' hair or in their bedding; when fresh or rehydrated, somewhat rectangular with a single lateral pore; eggs may be found on fecal flotation; eggs are brown, slightly oval, up to 49 μm (depending on species) in size, shell has radial striations; cannot be differentiated from those of *Echinococcus* spp. (Figure 5–2).

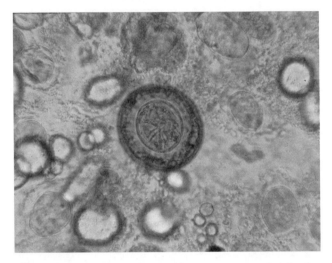

Figure 5–2 Cestode egg featured here was recovered on fecal flotation from a dog. It is probably *Taenia*, but could also be *Echinococcus* (600×).

POSTMORTEM

- Definitive hosts: tapeworms may be up to 2 m in length; scolex with four suckers, armed rostellum with two rows of hooks; mature and gravid segments rectangular, single-pored; lives in small intestine.

- Intermediate hosts: finding metacestodes in characteristic sites is usually enough to suggest the most likely species involved; definitive identification requires specialist.

Treatment and Control

- See Tables 4–5 and 4–6 for treatment.

- Prevent scavenging and predation by dogs or cats whenever possible; do not feed raw meat.

ECHINOCOCCUS SPP.

- Includes *Echinococcus granulosus* and *E. multilocularis*; moderate significance to veterinary medicine but highly significant to public health.

- Distribution of *E. granulosus* includes North and South America, England, Africa, the Middle East, Australia, and New Zealand; distribution of *E. multilocularis* includes north-central Europe, Japan, Alaska, Canada, and the central United States.

Life Cycle

- Indirect.

- See Table 5–1 for intermediate host spectrum.

- Metacestode: hydatid cyst; develops in approximately 5 months for *E. granulosus* and 2–3 months for *E. multilocularis*; cysts may die or persist for the life of the intermediate host.

- *Echinococcus granulosus* produces unilocular cysts characterized by a thick, multilayered cyst wall with a thin, internal germinal membrane; protoscolices and daughter cysts, containing more protoscolices, may form internally; cysts are contained by a connective tissue capsule and do not invade surrounding tissue; *E. multilocularis* produces a multilocular cyst characterized by a thinner cyst wall; daughter cysts bud from the germinal layer and infiltrate surrounding tissue.

- For every hydatid cyst ingested by the definitive host, many tapeworms can develop.

- Prepatent period for *E. granulosus* is approximately 7 weeks and approximately 4 weeks for *E. multilocularis.*

Pathogenesis and Clinical Signs

- Adult tapeworms in carnivore definitive host are usually nonpathogenic.

- Hydatid cysts in the rodent and ungulate intermediate hosts appear to be well tolerated with clinical signs usually only in older animals; hydatid cysts in humans can cause signs of liver dysfunction or respiratory disease; if cyst ruptures, anaphylaxis results.

Diagnosis

ANTEMORTEM

- Definitive hosts only: eggs may be found on fecal flotation; eggs are brown, slightly oval, up to 40 µm in size, shell has radial striations; cannot be differentiated from those of *Taenia* spp. (see Figure 5–2); a coproantigen test kit is commercially available in Germany; because of their small size, gravid segments are generally overlooked when shed with feces.

POSTMORTEM

- Definitive hosts: very small tapeworms, 2–7 mm long, scolex with four suckers, armed rostellum with two rows of hooks; lives in small intestine; definitive identification requires specialist. Note: because of the serious zoonotic potential of these parasites, extreme caution is required in handling suspect material.

- Intermediate hosts: finding hydatid cyst is enough to diagnose echinococcosus.

Treatment and Control

- See Table 4–5 for treatment.
- Prevent scavenging and predation by dogs and cats whenever possible.

MONIEZIA SPP.

- Worldwide distribution in ruminants; low to moderate significance in adult animals, may be highly significant in young.

Life Cycle

- Indirect.
- Intermediate hosts: oribatid mites.
- Metacestode: cysticercoid; develops in approximately 4 months after mite ingests hexacanth embryo.
- Prepatent period is 4–7 weeks; lives approximately 3 months.
- Lambs and calves begin acquiring infections at the start of grazing.
- A seasonality exists in the release of eggs and/or proglottids; in temperate zones, it begins in May, peaks in June, and rapidly declines thereafter.

Pathogenesis and Clinical Signs

- Generally asymptomatic in light infections.
- Substantial numbers in lambs and kids may cause digestive disorders, diarrhea, cachexia; death may occur, but is rare.

Diagnosis

ANTEMORTEM

- Proglottids, which are wider than long, may be found in feces.
- Eggs are of typical anoplocephalid type (Figure 5–3); can be found using standard fecal flotation procedures.
- *Moniezia benedeni* eggs are square, approximately 75 μm in diameter.

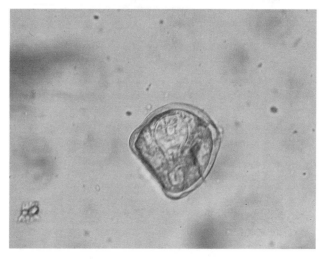

Figure 5-3 Cestode egg featured here is typical anoplo-cephalid-type that is representative of *Moniezia, Anoplocephala,* and *Paranoplocephala* (400×).

- *Moniezia expansa* eggs are triangular, 56–67 µm in diameter.

POSTMORTEM

- *Moniezia benedeni*: up to 4 m in length and 25 mm in width; scolex with four prominent suckers, without rostellum or hooks; segments wider than long; interproglottidal glands at the posterior margin of segments occupy midzone of segment (seen in stained specimens only); lives in small intestine.

- *Moniezia expansa*: up to 6 m in length and 15 mm in width; scolex with four prominant suckers, without rostellum or hooks; segments wider than long; interproglottidal glands at the posterior margin of segments extend the full width of the segment (seen in stained specimens only); lives in small intestine.

Treatment and Control

- See Table 4–3 for treatment.
- Prevent pasture contamination by a strategic treatment in the spring; reduction of mites on pasture impractical.

Small and Large Intestines, Cecum

ANOPLOCEPHALA PERFOLIATA, A. MAGNA, AND PARANOPLOCEPHALA MAMILLANA

- Worldwide distribution in equids; *A. perfoliata* most common.

Life Cycle

- Indirect.

- Intermediate hosts: oribatid mites.

- Metacestode: cysticercoid; develops approximately 4 months after mite ingests hexacanth embryo.

- Prepatent period is 4–8 weeks.

Pathogenesis and Clinical Signs

- *Anoplocephala magna* and *P. mamillana* not usually considered to be pathogenic.

- Attachment of *A. perfoliata* causes damage to intestinal mucosa that tends to increase in severity with increasing numbers of cestodes.

- Lesions vary from slight mucosal congestion with raised focal ulceration to mucosal thickening with ulcers and nodular swellings at site of attachment to granulomatous lesions projecting into the lumen at the ileocecal junction.

- Inflammation, combined with change in bowel diameter at the ileocecal junction (common attachment site) may predispose to intussusception.

- Clinical signs include those of colic; less severe clinical signs include general unthriftiness, intermittent diarrhea, and weight loss.

Diagnosis

ANTEMORTEM

- Eggs are of typical anoplocephalid type (see Figure 5–3); difficult to find on fecal flotation due to sporadic shedding of proglottids/eggs; repeated fecal flotations using saturated sugar may be necessary.

- *Anoplocephala perfoliata* eggs are thick-walled, round to "D" shaped, 65–80 µm in diameter.

- *Anoplocephala magna* eggs similar to *A. perfoliata* but smaller (50–60 µm).

- *Paranoplocephala mamillana* eggs are thin-walled, oval, approximately 50 × 37 µm.

POSTMORTEM

- *Anoplocephala perfoliata*: 4–8 cm in length, up to 1.2 cm in width; scolex robust, with four prominent suckers, without rostellum or hooks, with flap of tissue (lappet) posterior to each sucker; segments wider than long; lives in terminal ileum, cecum, large intestine, particularly near ileocecal junction.

- *Anoplocephala magna*: 20–80 cm in length, up to 2.5 cm in width; scolex robust, with four prominent suckers, without rostellum, hooks, or lappets; segments wider than long; lives in jejunum.

- *Paranoplocephala mamillana*: 0.6–5 cm in length, up to 0.6 mm in width; scolex narrow, with four suckers, without rostellum, hooks, or lappets; segments wider than long; lives in proximal small intestine.

Treatment and Control

- Pyrantel pamoate at 13.2 mg base per kg is effective; daily administration of pyrantel tartrate at 2.64 mg per kg removes tapeworms and prevents reinfection.
- Prophylactic treatments will prevent and control infections by reducing pasture contamination; isolate new arrivals and treat prior to turn-out on pasture.

Cestodes, Pseudophyllidea

Small Intestine

SPIROMETRA MANSONOIDES

- Distribution includes North and South America in bobcats, raccoons, dogs, and cats; minor significance.

Life Cycle

- Indirect.
- First intermediate host: copepod.
- Second intermediate host: water snakes and frogs most likely, although any vertebrate group except fish can fill this role; plerocercoid that develops is called a sparganum.
- Paratenic host: any vertebrate group except fish; includes raccoons, cats, dogs, and humans.
- Prepatent period is 10–30 days.

Pathogenesis and Clinical Signs

- Definitive host: usually inapparent; may cause intermittent diarrhea.

- Second intermediate host: may cause subcutaneous lumps that migrate over time; eventually, spargana die, calcify, and are enclosed in a fibrous capsule.

Diagnosis

ANTEMORTEM

- In the definitive host, eggs are released through the uterine pore, rather than by detaching segments; once eggs have been discharged, several senile segments may be passed in feces together; because segments are intermittently passed, they are often missed by the owner and practitioner.

- Eggs may be found on fecal flotation.

- Eggs are ovoid, operculated, 60–65 × 35–37 μm, pointed at both ends; may be confused with fluke eggs.

POSTMORTEM

- Definitive host: slightly pinkish tapeworms up to 75 cm in length, scolex with two bothria, gravid segments with central uterine pore and spiraled uterus; found in the small intestine.

- Second intermediate host: sparganosis is provisionally identified upon finding the ribbon-like, whitish spargana (plerocercoids) within the musculature or subcutis.

Treatment and Control

- A single dose of praziquantel at 20 mg per kg is effective.
- Prevent predation and scavenging by dogs and cats whenever possible.

DIPHYLLOBOTHRIUM LATUM

- Distribution includes central Finland, central Europe, Italy, Japan, regions of the Baltic Sea and Volga Basin, and the northern United States.
- Common name: broad fish tapeworm.

Life Cycle

- Indirect.
- First intermediate host: copepod.
- Second intermediate host: freshwater fishes; heaviest infections in large, predatory fishes such as pike, walleye, and trout.
- Paratenic hosts: large, predatory fishes.
- Definitive host: domestic dog and cat, human, pig, bear, and other fish-eating mammals.
- Prepatent period is 21–28 days.

Pathogenesis and Clinical Signs

- Usually inapparent in all but humans where it can cause pernicious anemia.

Diagnosis

ANTEMORTEM

- In the definitive host, eggs are released through the uterine pore, rather than by detaching segments; once eggs have been discharged, several senile segments may be passed in feces together; because segments are intermittently passed, they are often missed by the owner and practitioner.

- Eggs may be found on fecal flotation.

- Eggs are ovoid, operculated, 67–71 × 40–51 μm, yellowish, rounded at both ends; may be confused with fluke eggs.

POSTMORTEM

- Definitive host: 1.5–4 m in length, scolex with two bothria, segments wider than long, gravid segments with central uterine pore and rosette-shaped uterus; found in the small intestine.

Treatment and Control

- Praziquantel at 35 mg per kg orally has been effective.

- Freeze fish at −10°C for 72 hours or cook adequately to kill larvae; do not feed raw fish to pets; prevent scavenging and predation by pets whenever possible.

Trematodes

Small Intestine

NANOPHYETUS SALMINCOLA

- Distribution limited to Pacific Northwest region of North America and eastern Siberia; definitive hosts include raccoon, mink, fox, coyote, dog, cat, and human.
- Common name: salmon poisoning fluke.

Life Cycle

- Indirect.
- First intermediate host: aquatic snails.
- Second intermediate host: numerous species of fish; salmonid fish most susceptible; metacercariae found primarily in kidneys, but also muscles and other parts of the body; infective within 10 days; may survive 5 or more years.
- Extra-intestinal migration does not occur in the definitive host.
- Prepatent period: 5–8 days.

Pathogenesis and Clinical Signs

- Second intermediate hosts.

  Fish can tolerate large numbers of metacercariae; however, can be highly pathogenic if rate of acquisition is rapid.

Renal edema, hemorrhagic areas in skin (due to invading cercariae), and obstructive and mechanical injury to heart muscle, retina, kidney tubules, pancreatic tissue, and gallbladder may occur.

Signs may include exophthalmia, decreased or erratic swimming activity.

- Dogs.

    Flukes may produce hemorrhagic enteritis, although rarely cause disease.

    Importance is in the transmission of *Neorickettsia helminthoeca*, the cause of "salmon-poisoning disease."

    The rickettsial organism is transovarially transmitted and is found in all developmental stages of the fluke.

    The disease is restricted to canids; clinical signs appear 6–10 days postingestion; signs include a sudden onset of fever accompanied by marked vomiting, diarrhea (may be hemorrhagic), ocular discharge, and lymphadenopathy.

    Mortality is 50–90%.

Diagnosis

ANTEMORTEM

- Fluke infection—identification of eggs on fecal flotation or sedimentation; eggs are 64–97 × 34–55 μm, yellowish brown with indistinct operculum.

- Rickettsial infection—based on combination of clinical signs compatible with the disease and demonstration of fluke eggs in feces (disease is not transmitted without the fluke being present).

POSTMORTEM
- Parasites are white, extremely small, 0.5–2.0 mm in length; live in small intestine; because of small size, detection of the fluke may require scraping gut and checking material under a microscope.

Treatment and Control
- Praziquantel at 7–38 mg per kg given SQ or IM is effective.
- Prevent scavenging and predation by dogs whenever possible; do not feed raw fish to dogs.

ALARIA SPP.
- Several species in wild carnivores in South America, Europe, Africa, Australia, and northern North America; occasionally dogs; minor significance.

Life Cycle
- Indirect.
- First intermediate host: freshwater snails.
- Second intermediate host: tadpoles.
- Paratenic host: mice, rats, snakes, birds, humans.

- Definitive host becomes infected by ingesting the second intermediate or paratenic host; immature fluke migrates through the abdominal and thoracic cavities to lungs or arrives in lungs via the circulation; flukes migrate up the trachea, are swallowed, and mature in the small intestine.
- Prepatent period: 3–5 weeks.

Pathogenesis and Clinical Signs

- Generally asymptomatic; heavy infections may be associated with a catarrhal enteritis; human death resulting from massive fluke migrations has been recorded.

Diagnosis

ANTEMORTEM

- Eggs may be found in feces with either flotation or sedimentation technique; sedimentation does not distort eggs whereas flotation media can.
- Eggs are ovoid, operculated, dark yellow, 98–134 × 62–68 μm.

POSTMORTEM

- Parasites are small, 2–6 mm in length, with a flat, expanded anterior half and cylindrical posterior half; found in the small intestine.

Treatment and Control

- Praziquantel at 20 mg per kg is effective.
- Prevent predation and scavenging whenever possible.

6

Parasites of the Gastrointestinal Tract III–Protozoans

Apicomplexans
Small and Large Intestines

EIMERIA SPP.

- Worldwide distribution in rodents, lagomorphs, ruminants, pigs, birds, occasionally horses; high significance.

- Numerous species described including *Eimeria bovis*, *E. zuernii*, *E. auburnensis*, *E. alabamensis*, and *E. ellipsoidalis* of cattle; *E. ahsata, E. ovinoidalis,* and *E. ovina* in sheep; *E. arloingi, E. alijevi,* and *E. christenseni* in goats; *E. scabra* in pigs; *E. tenella, E. brunetti,*

E. acervulina, and *E. necatrix* in chickens; *E. melea-grimitis, E. adenoeides,* and *E. gallopavonis* in turkeys; *E. leuckarti* in horses.

- High degree of host specificity, although a few species can infect other related hosts.

Life Cycle

- Direct.

- Each cycle has several asexual generations and one sexual generation.

- Unsporulated oocysts are passed in the feces; becomes infective through a process called sporulation; each zygote divides into four cells; each cell forms a sporocyst; each sporocyst develops two sporozoites within; sporozoites are infective stage.

- Infection is acquired by ingestion of sporulated oocysts; sporozoites are released and penetrate the intestinal wall; each species enters a specific type of host cell; reproduce asexually forming meront (= schizont) containing merozoites (individual parasites); growing meronts destroy host cells and release merozoites that penetrate new cells; each species undergoes a set number of meront generations (usually 2, can be 3 or 4); merozoites then penetrate new host cells and enter sexual phase; produce male and female gamonts called microgametes and macrogametes, respectively; microgametes leave cell to fertilize macrogametes; fertilized macrogametes become oocysts; oocysts break out of host cell to be passed in the feces.

- Prepatent period is 4–22 days, depending on species.

- Because each species has a set number of asexual generations and a single sexual generation, infections are said to be self-limiting.

- Ingestion of a single sporulated oocyst can result in production of several hundred thousand oocysts.

Pathogenesis and Clinical Signs

- Not all species are equally pathogenic; severity of disease depends on the species present and the number of oocysts ingested; if low numbers are ingested, disease is usually not apparent and immunity produced with repeated infections; if moderate numbers are ingested, disease is usually mild and immunity produced; if large numbers are ingested, disease is usually severe and death may result; immunity is species-specific and incomplete.

- Destruction of host cells is the primary pathogenic mechanism; clinical signs include a severe, sometimes bloody, diarrhea and rapid loss of condition; death may occur during the prepatent period; survivors suffer long-term negative effects on growth rate; disease occurs most commonly in young animals and tends to be associated with stress: parturition, weaning, shipping, feed changes, adverse weather, intensive animal husbandry.

- Cattle: infection is common but disease is sporadic; usually calves <1 year old; light infections cause soft to watery feces and reduced weight gain; severe infections cause projectile bloody diarrhea containing mucus, rectal tenesmus, inappetence, dehydration, and weight loss; signs last approximately 1 week.

- Sheep: infection is common but disease is usually limited to lambs <6 months old; clinical signs as for cattle, but blood and tenesmus usually not present.

- Goats: infection is common with disease occurring in kids >2 weeks old; especially prevalent 2–3 weeks after weaning; clinical signs include pasty, watery diarrhea and dehydration.

- Pigs: infections are common but disease is not; *Isospora suis* responsible for neonatal porcine coccidiosis (see next section).

- Horses: prevalence unknown; infections usually inapparent.

- Chickens: infections are a major problem for the industry due to lost production; severe disease usually occurs in 3–6-week-old chicks; infections may be inapparent or signs of poor growth; sudden appearance of mucoid diarrhea (may be bloody) or death may occur; recovery in 1–2 weeks but adverse effects on production continue.

Diagnosis

ANTEMORTEM
- Unsporulated oocysts may be found on fecal flotation; presence or absence of oocysts does not necessarily correlate with presence of disease.

- Oocysts generally medium to large size (>12 µm; Figure 6–1); those of *E. leuckarti* are unusually large (80–88 × 55–59 µm) and require flotation media with higher specific gravity or the use of sedimentation to recover them; most species can be distinguished on basis of morphological features; however, most practitioners usually do not differentiate species.

POSTMORTEM

- May see developmental stages in histological sections of affected intestinal tract.
- In chickens, gross lesions in specific areas of the intestinal tract may be diagnostic.

Treatment and Control

- Because available drugs target early asexual stages, ability to treat infections is limited; treatment may consist of supportive therapy only; resistance to many compounds occurs, especially in coccidia of poultry; minimize exposure of other animals to oocysts and stressful conditions.
- Cattle: amprolium, monensin, or sulfa drugs (e.g., sulfamethazine) for treatment; amprolium, decoquinate, lasalocid, and monensin for prophylaxis.
- Sheep: decoquinate, lasalocid, and sulfaquinoxaline for prophylaxis.
- Goats: decoquinate and monensin for prophylaxis.

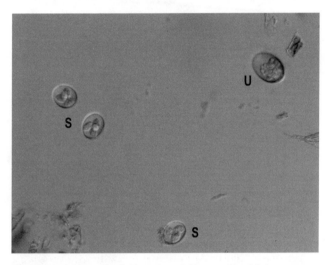

Figure 6–1 Sporulated (S) and partially sporulated (U) oocysts of *Eimeria* spp. (200×).

- Poultry: sulfa drugs, amprolium, monensin, and several others are available for prophylaxis.
- Young animals should be kept in clean, dry areas, not overcrowded or stressed; a live vaccine is available for use in chickens (breeders and layer replacements).

ISOSPORA SPP.

- Worldwide distribution in carnivores and pigs; low to moderate significance.
- Numerous species described including *Isospora canis* and *I. ohioensis* of dogs; *I. felis* and *I. rivolta* of cats; *I. suis* of pigs.
- Highly host specific.

Life Cycle

- Direct; indirect with paratenic host.
- Direct life cycle is similar to that of *Eimeria*; sporulation of oocysts passed in feces results in two sporocysts each containing four sporozoites per oocyst.
- Prepatent period is 4–11 days, depending on species.
- Indirect life cycle occurs in *I. canis* and *I. felis*; oocysts ingested by mice and birds; sporozoites penetrate small intestine, migrate to various organs, enlarge (do not reproduce), and encyst (now called hypnozoite); cat or dog becomes infected when ingesting infected paratenic host; importance of this route of transmission is unknown.
- Some authorities use the genus *Cystisospora* for those capable of developing in intermediate hosts.

Pathogenesis and Clinical Signs

- Similar to that described for *Eimeria*; destruction of host cells primary pathogenic mechanism; infections tend to be self-limiting.

- Carnivores: often inapparent; clinical signs of diarrhea, abdominal pain, dehydration, anorexia, and weight loss have been reported; disease associated with debilitated or very young hosts, massive infections or a particularly pathogenic strain of parasite.

- Pigs: causes neonatal porcine coccidiosis characterized by pale, watery, fetid diarrhea and decreased growth in piglets 5–15 days old; high morbidity and low mortality.

Diagnosis

ANTEMORTEM

- Unsporulated oocysts may be found on fecal flotation; presence or absence of oocysts does not necessarily correlate with presence of disease.

- Oocysts generally medium to large size (>12 μm); oocyts of *Isospora* of cats are larger than those of *Toxoplasma gondii*; oocysts of *I. suis* of pigs can be differentiated from those of *Eimeri* spp. based on number of sporocysts and sporozoites within the oocyst.

POSTMORTEM

- Asexual and sexual stages can be seen in histological sections of affected intestinal tract.

Treatment and Control

- Dogs: sulfadimethoxine administered at 55 mg per kg for 1 day, then 27.5 mg per kg for 4 days or until the dog is without clinical signs for at least 2 days, has been used.

- Pigs: neonatal porcine coccidiosis is apparently nonresponsive to treatment; on farms known to be highly contaminated, can prophylactically treat sows for 2 weeks prior to farrowing or piglets for the first 3 weeks of life.

SARCOCYSTIS SPP.

- Worldwide distribution in canids and felids; generally low significance.

- Numerous species described (Table 6–1).

Life Cycle

- Indirect.

- Free sporocysts or sporulated oocysts containing two sporocysts with four sporozoites are passed in the feces; ingested by the intermediate host; sporozoites enter vascular endothelial cells and undergo two meront generations; merozoites then invade skeletal and cardiac muscles and produce sarcocysts containing several hundred to thousands of bradyzoites; development to infective stage requires 1–2 months.

Table 6–1   Species of *Sarcocystis* Encountered in Veterinary Medicine

Species of *Sarcocystis*	Intermediate Host	Definitive Host
S. cruzi	Cattle	Dog, coyote, fox, wolf, raccoon, jackal
S. hirsuta		Cat
S. hominis		Humans, primates
S. tenella	Sheep	Dog, coyote, fox
S. arieticanis		Dog
S. gigantea		Dog
S. capracanis	Goat	Dog, coyote, fox
S. miescheriana	Pig	Dog, fox, raccoon, jackal
S. porcifelis		Cat
S. suihominis		Humans, primates
S. fayeri	Horse	Dog
S. bertrami		Dog
S. neurona	Unknown	Opossum*

Sarcocystis neurona is presented in Chapter 8.

- Definitive host acquires infection when ingesting bradyzoites; bradyzoites penetrate cells of the small intestine, form micro- and macrogametes; oocysts develop after fertilization.
- Prepatent period approximately 14 days, depending on species.

Pathogenesis and Clinical Signs

- Generally nonpathogenic for definitive host.
- Pathogenicity varies for intermediate host; species with canid definitive hosts generally more pathogenic than those with felid definitive hosts.
- Disease uncommon; naturally occurring clinically acute disease has only been reported in cattle; clinical signs usually associated with second generation meronts in the blood vessels; signs may include fever, inappetence, anemia (normocytic, normochromic), emaciation, abortion, death.

Diagnosis

ANTEMORTEM
- Definitive host: sporulated oocysts or free sporocysts may be found on fecal flotation; oocysts are dumbbell-shaped, 15–20 × 12–16 µm in size, with thin oocyst wall; sporocysts are 12–15 × 8–10 µm.
- Intermediate host: difficult and not usually attempted by the practitioner.

POSTMORTEM

- Intermediate host: generally by finding sarcocysts in skeletal or cardiac tissue in histologic section.

Treatment

- Generally do not treat domestic animals for infection.

- Control in intermediate host consists of eliminating fecal contamination of feed; elevate feed and water troughs to prevent feeding off contaminated ground.

- Practical control in definitive host consists of eliminating raw or undercooked meat from the diet.

TOXOPLASMA GONDII

- Worldwide distribution in domestic and wild felids; moderate significance to veterinary medicine; may be highly significant to public health.

Life Cycle

- Indirect with paratenic host or direct.

- Unsporulated oocysts are passed in feces; sporulate to infective oocysts within approximately 24 hours; oocysts contain two sporocysts each with four sporozoites; infective to virtually all warm-blooded animals; in paratenic host, sporozoites invade intestinal cells and associated lymph nodes to become rapidly dividing tachyzoites; rupture cells, spread throughout the body, encyst, and form bradyzoites.

- Paratenic host can also be infected by ingesting bradyzoites; these form tachyzoites and the cycle repeats as before.

- Only felids are definitive hosts; become infected by ingesting either tissue cysts containing infective bradyzoites (most common route) or oocysts; bradyzoites or sporozoites invade epithelial cells of the small intestine, undergoing several asexual generations ending with production of micro- and macrogametes and oocysts.

- Prepatent period is 3–10 days if tissue cysts are source of infection and 19–21 days if oocysts are source of infection; excrete oocysts for only 1–2 weeks.

- Felids can also harbor tissue cysts.

- Transplacental transmission can occur if dam is infected during pregnancy; tachyzoites migrate to fetus; congenital infections important for humans, sheep, and goats.

Pathogenesis and Clinical Signs

- Varies with the host, route of infection, immune status, and organ affected.

- Cats: infections are usually inapparent; clinical infections most commonly associated with pneumonia.

- Sheep and goats: infection of dam during pregnancy may result in abortion, macerated or mummified feti, stillbirths, or perinatal mortality; infection may also be fatal in adult goats.

- Pigs: infection in adults is usually inapparent, but pregnant sows may abort or give premature birth; in piglets (<12 weeks old), infections may be associated with fever, pneumonia, myocarditis, and encephalitis.

- Dogs: clinical disease uncommon; usually occurs concurrently with canine distemper virus infection and involves the lungs, liver, and CNS.

- Humans: infections occur primarily through ingestion of undercooked meat although oocysts may also cause infections; chorioretinitis most common sequelae of congenital infection but hydrocephalus, mental retardation, and jaundice may also occur; an estimated 1 in 1,000 children are born infected with *T. gondii* in the United States.

Diagnosis

ANTEMORTEM
- Felids: unsporulated oocysts may be found on fecal flotation; oocysts are subspherical, 10×12 µm; cannot distinguish *T. gondii* oocysts from those of *Hammondia hammondi*, another coccidian parasite of cats, without experimental life cycle studies, so all 10×12 µm oocysts should be considered *T. gondii* unless proven otherwise; serologic tests are available, but need to measure both IgM and IgG and/or do paired serum tests.

- Paratenic hosts: may be able to demonstrate organisms on stained impression smear of lymph node biopsy.

POSTMORTEM

- Demonstration of *anti-T. gondii* IgM antibodies in goat, sheep, or pig fetus indicates infection because IgM does not cross the placenta in ruminants and pigs.

- May find organism in histologic sections of enlarged lymph nodes or other lesions.

- Other techniques (i.e., isolation of organism from infected tissue in mice or tissue culture) are available from specialized laboratories.

Treatment and Control

- Generally do not treat domestic animals for infection.

- Clinically ill cats can be treated with clindamycin hydrochloride; begin with 25 mg per kg, twice daily, orally with food and progress to 50 mg per kg, twice daily; treat for a minimum of 2 weeks.

- Control in the domestic cat consists of confining the animal indoors to prevent hunting and feeding the cat only commercially prepared cat food.

- Control in humans is achieved by cooking all meats to at least 70°C and washing hands and utensils with soap and water; cat litter should be emptied daily to remove oocysts before they sporulate; cat pan should be rinsed with boiling water; wear rubber gloves when gardening; wash raw vegetables thoroughly.

NEOSPORA SPP.

- Includes *Neospora caninum* of cattle, dogs, sheep, goats, and horses, and *N. hughesi* of horses; serologic evidence for human exposure to *N. caninum* exists.
- Worldwide distribution.

Life Cycle

- Indirect.
- Details are incomplete; dogs can be both intermediate and definitive host; cattle, sheep, and goats are intermediate hosts.
- Tachyzoites and tissue cysts with bradyzoites are found in the intermediate host; cysts tend to be found primarily in CNS, but also in peripheral nerves and retina.
- Thought that dogs acquire infection by ingesting tissue cysts; shed unsporulated oocysts that sporulate within 72 hours; each oocysts contains two sporocysts with four sporozoites.
- Congenital transmission also occurs.

Pathogenesis and Clinical Signs

- Primary pathogenic mechanism may be cellular destruction resulting from multiplication of the tachyzoites.
- Cattle: a primary cause of abortion in dairy cattle in the United States; any age cow may abort from 3 months

gestation to term with most occurring mid-gestation (5–6 months); cows do not need to acquire infection during pregnancy to abort and may abort repeatedly; congenitally infected calves may be underweight, unable to rise, and present with signs of CNS disorders; reduced milk production in first-lactation heifers can occur in chronically infected animals.

- Dogs: disease is most severe in congenitally infected pups, but fatal infections have been reported in dogs 8–15 years old; dogs are bright, alert, and present with an ascending paralysis; hind limbs more often affected than front limbs; other clinical signs may include paralysis of the jaw, muscle flaccidity or atrophy; dermatitis in adult dogs may occur.

- Goats: abortions have been reported in pygmy goats and dairy goats.

- Sheep: experimental infections will induce abortion, but reports of natural cases are rare.

- Horses: infections have various manifestations ranging from apparent abortion to CNS disorders; whether *N. hughesi* or *N. caninum* is primarily responsible for disease is unclear.

Diagnosis

ANTEMORTEM

- Antibodies against *N. caninum* can be detected with various serological tests, many of which are available at specialized laboratories; interpret with caution—in cattle, a negative test for an aborted cow can exclude *N. caninum* as the cause of abortion in individual cows; a positive serologic test for an aborted cow or fetus indicates only infection, not abortion; a negative serologic test for a fetus does not rule out infection.

- Although naturally infected dogs have yet to be identified as shedding oocysts, be on the lookout for unsporulated oocysts in feces that are spherical to subspherical and 10–11 μm in diameter; must be differentiated from *Isospora*.

POSTMORTEM

- May find tissue cysts on histological section; tissue cysts of *N. hughesi* are smaller than those of *N. caninum*, have thinner cyst walls (≤ 1 μm) and smaller bradyzoites; immunohistochemical staining required for definitive diagnosis.

Treatment and Control

- Currently, there is no effective treatment.
- Control may presumably be achieved by eliminating fecal contamination of feed and water by dogs.

CRYPTOSPORIDIUM SPP.

- Worldwide distribution in mammals (including humans), fish, reptiles, and birds; highly significant to veterinary medicine and public health.

- Includes *C. parvum* of mammals (including humans), *C. muris* of rodents and possibly cattle, *C. andersoni* of cattle, *C. baileyi* and *C. meleagridis* of chickens and turkeys; based on molecular analyses, more species probably exist.

Life Cycle

- Direct.
- Sporulated oocysts are passed with the feces; after ingestion, sporozoites invade microvillous border of gastric glands, lower half of the small intestine, bile duct, or respiratory tract; lie in a vacuole just beneath the host cell membrane (intracellular but extracytoplasmic); undergo two or three meront generations (species dependent) followed by asexual development and oocyst production within 72 hours; oocysts sporulate before leaving the cells; two types of oocysts produced—thin-walled that break and reinfect the host, and thick-walled that pass in the feces.
- Prepatent period can be as short as 3 days.
- Oocysts are extremely resistant to environmental conditions and most man-made chemicals.

Pathogenesis and Clinical Signs

- Transmission among people or animals is by fecal contamination; infection may occur in any age animal but disease is usually limited to the very young (≤ 3 weeks old) or the immunocompromised.

- Pathogenesis not completely understood; little tissue reaction occurs as a result of the parasite; the parasite may decrease disaccharidase activity resulting in reduced breakdown of sugars resulting in bacterial overgrowth, formation of volatile fatty acids, and changes in osmotic pressure; these changes then cause the characteristic severe, watery diarrhea.

- *C. parvum*: disease is self-limiting, lasting 1–3 weeks in otherwise healthy animals; lesions present are mild to moderate villous atrophy, changes in surface epithelium and shortening of microvilli; severity of disease is exacerbated in the presence of other pathogens (e.g., rotavirus in calves).

- *C. andersoni* (possibly *C. muris*): infects the abomasum; clinically mild with possible adverse affects on weight gain and milk production; generally found in older cattle.

- *C. baileyi*: may infect bursa of Fabricius (BF), cloaca or respiratory tract of chickens, turkeys, ducks; the disease usually manifests as respiratory disease in chicks < 11 weeks old with intestinal disease less common; results in air sacculitis, pneumonia, sinusitis, conjunctivitis; clinical signs of respiratory infection include coughing, sneezing, dyspnea, rales; severity of disease is exacerbated in the presence of other pathogens (e.g., infectious bronchitis virus); infection of BF may diminish humoral immune response to vaccines.

- *C. meleagridis*: infects BF, cloaca, or respiratory tract of chickens and turkeys; disease apparently only occurs in turkeys.

Diagnosis

ANTEMORTEM
- Detection methods include:

    Fecal flotation—centrifugal or simple flotation; saturated sugar recommended (specific gravity of 1.33).

    Direct normal saline smear—can be air dried and stained with one of several methods to help visualize oocysts; not as good as fecal flotation.

    ELISA test—several test kits commercially available for humans; may be useful in other mammals; detects parasite antigen in feces; can be expensive.

    Immunofluorescence—numerous test kits commercially available; in general, better sensitivity and specificity than stained smears; however, requires immunofluorescent microscope.

- Oocysts are tiny, subspherical, 3–7 μm in diameter.

POSTMORTEM
- In addition to antemortem methods, may find developmental stages on histological section in microvillous border of affected tissue.

Treatment and Control

- Paromomycin has been shown capable of preventing clinical signs and mortality and decreasing oocysts output in calves, kids, and cats.

- Control is difficult; strict sanitation is needed; separation of susceptible animals from dams may be required including separate personnel to care for each.

Flagellates
Small Intestine

GIARDIA DUODENALIS

- Worldwide distribution in mammals, birds, and amphibians.

- Five species currently recognized including *Giardia duodenalis* in domestic and wild mammals (including humans) and *G. muris* in rodents; based on molecular analyses, more species may exist.

- Note: three names are given to the species that infects humans—*G. intestinalis*, *G. lamblia*, and *G. duodenalis*; based on the rules of zoological nomenclature, the name *G. lamblia* is without taxonomic basis and is invalid; however, either *G. duodenalis* or *G. intestinalis* can be used; *G. duodenalis* will be used here in keeping with the most recent proposal.

Life Cycle

- Direct.

- Transmitted by the fecal-oral route, primarily through feed and/or water contaminated with cysts; cysts are passed with the feces; each cyst contains two trophozoites; upon ingestion, trophozoites leave the cyst, attach to the brush border of the jejunum, and multiply through binary fission; subsequently, each trophozoite forms a cyst; asexual reproduction occurs resulting in two trophozoites within the cyst.

- Trophozoites can also be passed with the feces, particularly during acute infections, resulting in transmission of the parasite; however, cysts are more resistant to external environmental conditions and are the stage most often responsible for continued transmission.

- Prepatent period is 5–16 days.

- Infections are more common in young animals; are probably the most important source of environmental contamination; adults, especially dams, can be sources for their offspring; a periparturient rise in cyst excretion has been shown to occur in sheep.

Pathogenesis and Clinical Signs

- Infections have been shown to cause villous atrophy and crypt hyperplasia; this results in a decrease in the absorptive surface area of the small intestine; glucose, water, and sodium absorption is hindered.

- Decreased activity of disaccharidase also occurs, which impairs digestion.

- Ruminants—clinical signs are often absent; when present, they may include diarrhea and weight loss; impaired growth rate in lambs has been documented.

- Horses—clinical signs are often absent; have been associated with diarrhea, ill thrift, and reduced growth rate in foals.

- Dogs and cats—clinical signs are often absent; when present, they may include acute, chronic, or intermittent foul smelling, fatty diarrhea, vomiting, dehydration, anorexia.

Diagnosis

ANTEMORTEM

- Detection of trophozoite or cyst in feces; intermittent shedding makes diagnosis difficult; therefore, giardiosis should not be ruled out based on a single negative fecal exam; it is recommended three fecal examinations over a period of 7–10 days be performed.

- Detection methods include:

   Fecal flotation—centrifugal or simple flotation used to detect cysts; zinc sulfate usually listed as the recommended flotation medium, however, saturated sugar also works; diluted iodine added to prep allows for better visualization of morphology.

   Direct normal saline smear—best if performed within 20 minutes of sample collection; motile trophozoites detected in unstained prep; diluted iodine added to prep kills the organisms but allows for better visualization of morphology.

   ELISA test—several test kits commercially available for humans; may be useful in other mammals; detects parasite antigen in feces; can be expensive.

   Immunofluorescence—numerous test kits commercially available; detects cysts and/or trophozoites with fluorescent antibodies; in general, better sensitivity and specificity than iodine-stained smears; however, requires immunofluorescent microscope.

Duodenal aspiration—fluid is aspirated and the sediment examined for trophozoites; requires either endoscopy or laparotomy; usually only recommended if animal has not been treated, zinc sulfate flotation has not been performed, and the animal is undergoing upper gastrointestinal endoscopy.

- Trophozoites are pear-shaped, bilaterally symmetrical with a concave adhesive disc on the ventral surface, with two nuclei and four pairs of flagella, 9–21 × 5–15 μm; when stained, resemble a "clown face."

- Cysts are oval, with 2–4 nuclei and other elements characteristic of the trophozoites that they contain, 9–13 × 7–10 μm.

POSTMORTEM

- In addition to the antemortem detection methods, a direct saline smear of the scrapings of the small intestine can be used to detect trophozoite stages.

Treatment and Control

- Dogs: fenbendazole at the same dosage used for helminths has been used; metronidazole (22 mg per kg orally twice daily for 5 days) has also been effective; metronidazole is still the drug of choice followed by fenbendazole in the case of treatment failure.

- Cats: metronidazole as for dogs.

- Calves: fenbendazole at varying dosages (a single 10 mg dose, 10–20 mg per day for 3 days, 0.833 mg daily for 6 days) or albendazole at 20 mg per day for 3 days has been used.

- Because of the potential of transmission to humans, treatment of household pets is warranted; cysts survive best under cool, humid conditions so keeping areas dry is important; cysts are susceptible to quaternary ammonium solutions recommended for kennel disinfection so prompt removal of feces and frequent and thorough cleaning of kennels is recommended.

Upper Gastrointestinal Tract
TRICHOMONAS GALLINAE

- Widespread distribution in pigeons, doves, raptors, gallinaceous birds; moderate significance.

Life Cycle

- Direct.

- Avian host becomes infected by ingesting the parasite with feed, water, litter, regurgitated crop contents, or in the case of raptors, prey (e.g., doves).

Pathogenesis and Clinical Signs

- Causes an inflammation and ulceration of the mouth, sinuses, esophagus, crop, and proventriculus, which may extend to the liver, serosal surface of the intestinal tract, pancreas, and heart.

- Clinical signs include yellowish circumscribed

lesions or caseous nodules anywhere from the oro-cavity to proventriculus; caseous, greenish exudate may accumulate, exuding from the beak.

Diagnosis

ANTEMORTEM
- Parasites may be found on direct saline smear of crop contents; characterized by four anterior flagella.

POSTMORTEM
- Typical lesions may be found within the digestive tract, liver; direct saline smear of crop contents to demonstrate organisms.

Treatment and Control

- Can use metronidazole at 30–60 mg per kg orally, twice daily for 5–7 days; 10 mg of carnidazole orally in a single dose has been used in nonfood pigeons; resistance to both drugs has been reported.

- Minimize contact of poultry with pigeons or doves; raise birds on wire platforms to avoid fecal contamination; do not feed pigeons or doves to raptors in rehabilitation.

Ciliates
Colon

BALANTIDIUM COLI
- Worldwide distribution in pigs; rarely humans, other primates, rats, dogs.

Life Cycle

- Direct.
- Transmitted through the fecal-oral route via cysts or trophozoites; cysts more resistant to external environment.

Pathogenesis and Clinical Signs

- Generally nonpathogenic to pigs; may invade colonic mucosa if damaged by other pathogens.

Diagnosis

ANTEMORTEM

- May find trophozoites in direct smear of feces or cysts on fecal flotation.
- Trophozoites are oval, with funnel-shaped mouth, macronucleus and usually micronucleus, covered with cilia, 30–150 × 25–120 μm.
- Cysts are spherical, with double membrane, 40–60 μm.

POSTMORTEM

- In addition to antemortem techniques, may find trophozoites in histological sections of colonic tissue.

Treatment and Control

- Generally do not treat pigs for infection.
- To prevent human infections, use good hygiene.

7

Parasites of the Cardiopulmonary System

Nematodes

Respiratory Tract

DICTYOCAULUS SPP.

- Includes *D. viviparus* of cattle, *D. filaria* of sheep and goats, and *D. arnfieldi* of donkeys and horses.

- Worldwide distribution; *D. viviparus*—moderate significance, especially in dairy calves in temperate and moist regions of western and central Europe; in the United States, infections may be widespread, but disease is not; *D. filaria*—moderate to high significance, especially in young animals in eastern Europe, India, central and northeastern United States; *D. arnfieldi*—very common in donkeys, rare in horses.

Life Cycle

- Direct.
- *Dictyocaulus viviparus* and *D. filaria*: L_1 develops and hatches from eggs either in bronchi or the gastrointestinal tract; L_1 is passed in the feces; infective L_3 develops in 4–6 days.
- *Dictyocaulus arnfieldi*: L_1 hatches within a few hours of eggs being passed in the feces; infective L_3 develops in 3–7 days.
- Animals become infected by ingestion of infective L_3; larvae penetrate the small intestine, progress to the mesenteric lymph nodes, and molt to L_4; larvae continue to the lungs via the lymphatic and circulatory system, arriving there approximately 1 week after ingestion; they break out into the alveoli, molt to the adult stage, and mature.
- Prepatent period is 3–8 weeks, depending on species; larvae may arrest development, prolonging the prepatent period to 5 months.
- L_3 extremely susceptible to desiccation; rainy weather and damp or wet places in pastures favor development and survival; *D. viviparus* larvae do not migrate readily and rely on rain for dispersal.

Pathogenesis and Clinical Signs

- *Dictyocaulus viviparus*

    Larvae can cause inflammation anywhere in the lungs; alveoli may collapse or become epithelialized; clinical signs may include tachypnea, dyspnea, and a nonproductive cough.

    Adults can cause chronic bronchitis with affected lobes becoming consolidated as a result of fibrosis; clinical signs may include tachypnea, severe dyspnea, head extended in air hunger position, harsh cough, anorexia, weight loss, emaciation, death.

    Severity and duration of disease are related to how many and how fast larvae are ingested.

    Secondary bacterial infections and/or pulmonary edema and emphysema may occur.

    In temperate regions, disease usually occurs during the second half of the first grazing season in calves.

- *Dictyocaulus filaria*

    Causes a catarrhal bronchitis; exudate passes into alveoli leading to atelectasis or pneumonia; secondary bacterial infections may occur.

    Clinical signs include marked coughing, tachypnea, dyspnea, nasal discharge, weight loss, emaciation, death.

    Disease usually occurs during the second half of the first grazing season in lambs and kids.

- *Dictyocaulus arnfieldi*

    Patency usually only achieved in donkeys and mules; rare in horses.

    Donkeys are usually asymptomatic.

    Causes an eosinophilic pneumonitis in horses.

    Clinical signs may include chronic coughing, decreased exercise performance, general unthriftiness, respiratory distress.

Diagnosis

ANTEMORTEM

- *Dictyocaulus viviparus*: can detect L_1 in feces with the Baermann technique; use of flasks superior to funnels; can detect eggs and larvae in lavage fluid; larvae are 390–450 µm with a pointed tail and brown food granules in the intestinal cells.

- *Dictyocaulus filaria*: can detect L_1 in feces with the Baermann technique; larvae are 550–580 µm, with an anterior cuticular knob, blunt tail, and brown food granules in the intestinal cells.

- *Dictyocaulus arnfieldi*: usually cannot detect larvae in feces from affected horse; clinical signs and grazing history are the most helpful; can detect L_1 in feces from donkeys cograzing with affected animal with the Baermann technique; may also be able to detect eggs on fecal flotation if collected per rectum and examined quickly.

POSTMORTEM

- *Dictyocaulus viviparus* and *D. filaria*: parasites are white, up to 8 cm (*D. viviparus*) or 10 cm (*D. filaria*) in length; easy to recover from the trachea, bronchi, and bronchioles.

- *Dictyocaulus arnfieldi*: adults are white, up to 7 cm in length; found in smaller bronchioles in donkeys, mules; in horses, unlikely to find worms on gross necropsy because they do not tend to mature.

Treatment and Control

- Ruminants: see Table 4–3 for treatment; maintain adequate levels of nutrition; avoid overstocking and grazing of damp areas favoring larval survival; radiation-attenuated larval vaccines are commercially available in certain areas of Europe.

- Horses: possibly benzimidazoles or avermectins may be used; do not pasture donkeys and horses together.

MUELLERIUS CAPILLARIS

- Cosmopolitan distribution in small ruminants; locally abundant in areas of the United States; low to moderate significance, mostly in goats.

Life Cycle

- Indirect.
- Intermediate host: terrestrial snails and slugs.

- First-stage larvae develop and hatch from eggs laid in lungs, are coughed up, swallowed, and passed in the feces; penetrate snail or slug and develop to infective L_3 in approximately 2 weeks.

- Ruminant acquires infection by ingesting mollusc containing infective L_3; larvae are released from the mollusc, penetrate the intestine, and follow lymphatic system to right heart and lungs; enter alveoli and bronchioles and mature.

- Prepatent period is 38–48 days; parasites may undergo arrested development as immature adults, thereby prolonging the prepatent period.

Pathogenesis and Clinical Signs

- Usually inapparent.

- Infection associated with inflammation resulting in nodules that are granuloma-like areas containing mature worms, eggs, and L_1.

- Clinical signs may include dyspnea, coughing, and other signs of interstitial pneumonia.

Diagnosis

ANTEMORTEM

- Can detect L_1 in feces with Baermann technique; use of flasks is superior to funnels.

- Larvae are approximately 300 µm in length; larval tail with undulating tip and dorsal spine.

POSTMORTEM

- Finding typical pulmonary lesions at necropsy; may find nematodes in histological sections of affected lung.

Treatment and Control

- Generally do not treat for infection.

METASTRONGYLUS SPP.

- Worldwide distribution in pigs in outdoor management situations; also found in wild swine; moderate significance.

- Includes *M. apri*, *M. pudendotectus*, and *M. salmi*; mixed infections of *M. apri* and *M. pudendotectus* appear to be required for either to develop in the host.

Life Cycle

- Indirect.

- Intermediate host: earthworms.

- Fully larvated eggs are laid in lungs, coughed up, swallowed, and passed with the feces; earthworms ingest eggs; L_1 hatches in earthworm; infective L_3 present in 10–30 days.

- Pigs acquire infection by ingesting earthworms containing the infective L_3; larvae invade the small intestine, entering lymphatic vessels to reach the lungs by way of the right heart; molt to L_4 approximately 3 days postinfection in lymph nodes or lungs; molt to immature adult in lungs.

- Prepatent period is 3–6 weeks, depending on species; may live up to 6 months.

Pathogenesis and Clinical Signs

- Usually inapparent; disease, when present, occurs only in young pigs.
- Can cause bronchitis, hypersecretion of mucus, hypertrophy of the bronchiolar musculature, and emphysema leading to consolidation of the diaphragmatic lobes.
- Clinical signs primarily limited to coughing; may also include dyspnea, cyanosis, inappetence, weight loss, or decreased weight gain.

Diagnosis

ANTEMORTEM
- Eggs may be found on fecal flotation; eggs are dense and flotation medium should have a specific gravity of 1.25 or greater (e.g., saturated magnesium sulfate).
- Eggs are ellipsoidal, rough-shelled, 45–60 × 38–42 μm, each containing a larva.
- In older animals, egg shedding is intermittent and repeated fecal examinations may be necessary.

POSTMORTEM
- Adult worms are grayish white, 1.5–4.5 cm in length; found by squeezing the incised areas of consolida-

tion; species can be differentiated based on spicule morphology of the males.

Treatment and Control

- See Table 4–1 for treatment.
- Control by housing pigs, cultivating infected pasture, or cograzing with unsusceptible species of livestock.

SYNGAMUS TRACHEA

- Worldwide distribution in domestic fowl, game birds, ratites, raptors, passerine birds; moderate significance, especially in chicks, turkeys, pheasants, and partridges under range conditions.
- Common name: gapeworm.

Life Cycle

- Direct; indirect with paratenic host.
- Paratenic hosts: earthworms, slugs, beetles, and other arthropods.
- Eggs are laid in the trachea, coughed up, swallowed, and passed with the feces; L_1 develops to infective L_3 within the egg in 1–2 weeks; eggs may or may not hatch.
- Definitive host becomes infected by ingesting egg with infective L_3, L_3 after hatching, or paratenic host containing infective L_3; larvae migrate to the lungs via liver,

break out into alveoli, and molt to immature adult; migrate up bronchial tree to trachea and mature.

- Prepatent period is 17–21 days; may live up to 5 months in chickens and 7.5 months in turkeys.

- Chickens <10 weeks old are most susceptible; older birds can tolerate more nematodes than younger birds; infections tend to occur in summer when earthworms are active.

Pathogenesis and Clinical Signs

- Larval migration may cause petechial hemorrhages, inflammation, and edema; clinical signs may include dyspnea and depression.

- Adult parasites cause tracheitis, excess mucus production leading to partial occlusion of the airways, respiratory distress; adults also ingest blood leading to anemia; clinical signs may include coughing, weakness, emaciation, dyspnea, or signs of asphyxiation including open-mouthed breathing ("gaping"), death.

Diagnosis

ANTEMORTEM
- Eggs may be found on fecal flotation.

- Eggs are ellipsoidal, thin-shelled with nearly parallel sides, 70–100 × 43–46 μm, with a thickened operculum at each pole, containing morula with 8–16 cells.

POSTMORTEM

- The bright red female (0.5–3.0 cm in length) and smaller, white male (0.2–0.6 cm) live in permanent copulation appearing as the letter Y; found attached to the mucosa in the middle to distal parts of the trachea.

Treatment and Control

- Thiabendazole at 300–1500 mg per kg daily for 3 days is highly effective.
- Control by rearing chicks indoor to 4–5 weeks of age; separate chicks from adults; prevent contamination of yard by wild birds; keep yards dry.

AELUROSTRONGYLUS ABSTRUSUS

- Cosmopolitan distribution in cats; low to moderate significance.

Life Cycle

- Indirect.
- Intermediate hosts: snails and slugs.
- Paratenic hosts: small rodents, birds.
- Adult females deposit eggs in "nests" in the lung parenchyma; L_1 develops, hatches, is carried up the bronchial tree and trachea, swallowed, and passed in the feces; penetrate the intermediate host and develop to infective L_3 in 2–5 weeks.

- Ingestion of paratenic host is most probable route of infection for the cat; larvae migrate from the stomach to the lungs through the peritoneal and thoracic cavities.
- Prepatent period is 4–6 weeks.

Pathogenesis and Clinical Signs

- Many infections are inapparent; may cause sub-pleural nodules, smooth muscle hypertrophy of the bronchioles and alveolar ducts, bronchitis.
- Clinical signs may include coughing, dyspnea, sneezing, nasal discharge, inappetence.

Diagnosis

ANTEMORTEM

- L_1 may be found in feces using the Baermann technique.
- Larvae are 360–390 μm long with an S-curved tail bearing a subterminal spine.

POSTMORTEM

- Adult worms are long and slender, 0.5–1.0 cm in length, and easily missed in the lung tissue.

Treatment and Control

- Fenbendazole at 50 mg per kg daily for 3 days or a single SQ injection of ivermectin at 0.4 mg per kg is effective.

- Control is generally impractical without indoor confinement of animals.

EUCOLEUS BÖHMI
- Distribution unknown; moderate significance in domestic dogs.
- Common name: nasal capillarid.

Life Cycle
- Unknown.
- Most likely direct; earthworms may play a role in transmission as well.

Pathogenesis and Clinical Signs
- Parasites live in the epithelium of the nasal turbinates, frontal sinuses, and paranasal sinuses; epithelium becomes hyperemic and hyperplastic; excess mucus is produced.
- Clinical signs include sneezing, nasal discharge that may be bloody.

Diagnosis
ANTEMORTEM
- Eggs may be found in nasal discharge or on fecal flotation.
- Eggs are typical capillarid-type (see Figure 4–6), 54–60 × 30–35 µm, containing a multicellular embryo that

does not fill the egg; close examination reveals a delicately pitted surface; must be differentiated from other capillarid-type eggs that may be found in dogs.

- May find capillarid-type nematodes in nasal biopsy.

POSTMORTEM
- Because of their small size, these nematodes may be missed during gross necropsy; more likely to find capillarid-type nematodes in histologic section.

Treatment and Control
- A single oral dose of ivermectin at 0.2 mg per kg has been reported to be effective.

EUCOLEUS AEROPHILUS
- Worldwide distribution in felids, canids, and mustelids; generally of low significance.

Life Cycle
- Direct; indirect with earthworm.
- Eggs are laid in the lungs, coughed up, swallowed, and passed with the feces; L_1 develops, in 5–7 weeks, but does not hatch; eggs hatch if ingested by earthworm, but larvae do not develop further.
- Carnivore acquires infection by ingestion of infective eggs; larvae hatch in the intestine and migrate to lungs in 7–10 days.
- Prepatent period is approximately 40 days.

Pathogenesis and Clinical Signs

- Infections in domestic dogs and cats are, generally, inapparent.
- May cause bronchiole disease characterized by coughing and wheezing; secondary bacterial infections may occur.

Diagnosis

ANTEMORTEM
- Eggs may be found on fecal flotation.
- Eggs are capillarid-type (see Figure 4–6), 59–80 × 30–40 μm with a net-like pattern on the surface; must be differentiated from other capillarid-type eggs that may be present.

POSTMORTEM
- Adults live in the bronchi; generally do not see adult worms at necropsy; rather, usually find them on histologic sections.

Treatment and Control

- Fenbendazole at 50 mg per kg orally daily for 3 days may be effective.

Circulatory System

DIROFILARIA IMMITIS
- Distributed in tropical, subtropical, and warm temperate regions of the world in dogs, wild canids, cats, ferrets;

within the United States, endemic in all 50 states, but more common along the Atlantic and Gulf coasts, and the Mississippi River and its major tributaries.

- High significance to veterinary medicine; moderate significance to public health.
- Common name: heartworm.

Life Cycle

- Indirect.
- Intermediate host: mosquitoes.
- Adult females, living in pulmonary arteries/arterioles, produce microfilariae (mff); mosquito ingest mff with blood meal; develops to infective L_3 in 10–14 days.
- Definitive host becomes infected when mosquito containing the infective L_3 feeds; larvae escape from mouthparts to enter through the puncture wound left by mosquito; reside in skin and molts to L_4 within 10 days; migrates to muscle bundles and subcutaneous tissues where they reside for 2–3 months; molt to immature adult 60–70 days postinfection; migrate through venule walls and are carried to the heart and pulmonary arterioles by 3–4 months postinfection where they mature; may accidentally migrate to aberrant sites such as the brain and anterior chamber of the eye.
- Prepatent period is 6–9 months; adult can live 7+ years in dogs and 2–3 years in cats; mff can survive 2 years in dog's circulation.

- Transplacental transmission of mff has been reported.

- Larval development in mosquitoes does not occur when average daily temperature is below 17°C limiting the potential for heartworm transmission to 6 months or less in most of the continental United States.

Pathogenesis and Clinical Signs

- Dogs

    May be inapparent.

    Chronic heartworm disease: eosinophilic pneumonitis may occur; pulmonary endarteritis leads to proliferation of the intima and arterial hypertrophy; this favors thrombus formation and stenosis of the pulmonary artery; arteries lose elasticity; stenosis and loss of elasticity lead to persistent pulmonary hypertension that leads to right ventricular enlargement and chronic congestive heart failure; dead worms may form emboli that obstruct vessels; granulomatous reactions result; vessels are further occluded and infarcts develop; may be fatal; clinical signs may include chronic cough, dyspnea, peripheral edema, ascites, exercise intolerance.

    Vena cava or caval syndrome: in very heavy infections, worms may also reside in right heart and posterior vena cava; endocarditis, valvular insufficiency, venous stasis, and hemolysis occur; clinical signs are characterized by a sudden episode of profound lethargy and weakness, hemoglobinuria, dyspnea, tachycardia, icterus; fatal collapse occurs within 2–3 days.

Glomerulonephritis: occasional occurrence; a result of glomerular deposition of immune complexes involving mff.

- Cats

    May be inapparent.

    Harbor fewer worms than dogs (as few as two can be fatal); if infection becomes patent, mff are low in concentration and transient in the blood.

    Pathologic lesions similar to dogs; cats develop interstitial lung disease but rarely develop pulmonary hypertension and heart failure or caval syndrome.

    Clinical signs less specific than in dogs; may include coughing, intermittent vomiting usually unrelated to eating; occasional difficulty in breathing, panting, or open-mouth breathing; gagging, dyspnea, tachypnea, lethargy, anorexia, weight loss; death may occur suddenly, preceding clinical signs; clinical signs tend to be associated with either arrival of immature adults in the pulmonary arteries or death of mature worms resulting in thromboemboli and pulmonary arterial infarction and lung injury.

- Ferrets

    Infections probably under-recognized.

    May harbor only 1 worm and up to 30 worms; microfilaremia appears to be rare.

Infections may result in a severe pulmonary arteritis and an eosinophilic or granulomatous pneumonitis.

Clinical signs are similar to the dog but progress much more rapidly; signs include dyspnea, anorexia, holosystolic heart murmur, ascites, coughing, sudden death.

- Humans

   Numerous human cases have been reported; worms may reach the pulmonary artery but tend to die; results in pulmonary emboli and granuloma formation around pieces of dead worms; gives rise to coughing, dyspnea.

Diagnosis

ANTEMORTEM

- Dogs: antigen tests, which detect specific antigens from adult female worms, recommended as the first step; most tests detect infections that are 7–8 months old, infections with three (or sometimes fewer) mature female heartworms and are almost 100% specific; antigen tests generally do not detect infections of <5 months' duration, male-only infections, and are less accurate when <3 females are present; follow-up tests to detect mff in the blood are performed prior to chemotherapy; mff can be detected with wet mount of blood or with various concentration techniques (preferred) including the modified Knott's technique and filter tests; both concentrate and filter hemolyzed blood; must differentiate mff from those produced by *Acanthocheilonema reconditum* (Table 7–1).

- Cats: difficult; low worm numbers present are below detection limit of many antigen tests; tests also cannot detect infections with immature worms or infections with only male worms; antibody detection tests are available for screening cats for heartworm infection.

- Ferrets: antigen tests appear to be useful for detecting infections and can be used on thoracic or abdominal effusion as well.

POSTMORTEM
- Adult worms are white, slender, 12–30 cm in length; found in pulmonary arteries, possibly heart and posterior vena cava.

Treatment and Control

- Treatment is complicated and must be monitored carefully; dead and degenerating worms present post-treatment may worsen the clinical condition; treatment strategy consists of eliminating adults first, followed by elimination of mff if present, and then administration of preventives; the ivermectin monthly preventive has been shown to be capable of killing adult heartworms over prolonged periods of time.

- Melarsamine dihydrochloride and thiacetarsamide are approved for use in dogs to treat adult heart-

Table 7-1 Comparisons of Morphological and Other Characteristics of Microfilariae of *D. immitis* and *A. reconditum*

Characteristic	*Dirofilaria immitis*	*Acanthocheilonema reconditum*
Numbers present—wet mount	Numerous	Few
Motility—wet mount	Stationary	Progressive
Head shape—Knott, filter test	Tapered	Blunt
Tail—Knott test	Straight	Button hook
Body—Knott test	Straight	Curved
Length (µm)—wet smear	>310	<310
Length (µm)—Knott test	>275	<275
Length (µm)—filter test	>240	<240
Width (µm)—Knott test	>6.0	<6.0
Width (µm)—filter test	>5.8	<5.0

worms; after adulticide therapy, ivermectin at 0.05 mg per kg or milbemycin oxime at 0.5 mg per kg can be used to remove mff.

- Treatment in cats is even more complicated than in dogs; because the infection appears to be self-limiting, cats are often not treated or treated symptomatically.

- Treatment of ferrets is marginally successful as ferrets are at high risk of sudden death from worm emboli.

- Several preventives are available for both dogs and cats; ivermectin at 0.22 mg per kg has been used successfully in ferrets for prevention.

Trematodes
Respiratory Tract
PARAGONIMUS KELLICOTTI

- Eastern North American distribution in wild mammals, especially in the Mississippi River and tributaries; low to moderate significance in cats, dogs; may also occur in pigs.

Life Cycle

- Indirect.

- First intermediate host: aquatic or amphibious snails.

- Second intermediate host: crayfish; metacercariae released from dead crayfish remain viable up to 3 weeks.

- Paratenic host: rodents.

- Eggs are laid in the cysts within the lungs, pass through connecting channels to the bronchi, are coughed up, swallowed, and passed in the feces; miracidia develop in 2–7 weeks, hatch, and infect snails; cercariae are produced in 78–93 days, leave the snail, and infect the crayfish; metacercariae become infective in 42–46 days.

- Definitive host acquires infection by ingesting infected crayfish or metacercariae-contaminated water; metacercariae penetrate the intestine, migrate across the peritoneal cavity, penetrate the diaphragm and enter the lungs as early as 5 days postinfection; the flukes tend to pair up, form cysts, grow, and mature.

- Prepatent period is 30–36 days; may remain viable for up to 4 years.

Pathogenesis and Clinical Signs

- Infections may be inapparent.

- May cause eosinophilic peritonitis, pleuritis, and multifocal pleural hemorrhage during migratory phase.

- Chronic bronchiolitis, hyperplasia of bronchiole epithelium, and chronic eosinophilic granulomatous pneumonia associated with degenerating eggs; cyst rupture may lead to acute pneumothorax.

- Clinical signs may include intermittent coughing, dyspnea, lethargy.

Diagnosis

ANTEMORTEM

- Eggs may be found on fecal flotation or sedimentation; may also be found in direct smear of fluid obtained from lungs.

- Eggs are yellowish brown, 75–118 × 42–57 μm, with single operculum surrounded by distinct rim (Figure 7–1).

POSTMORTEM

- Worms are reddish brown, 7.5–16 mm in length; found in cysts within the lungs.

Treatment and Control

- Albendazole at 50 mg per kg daily for 21 days, fenbendazole at 50 mg per kg for 10–14 days, or praziquantel at 25 mg per kg 3 times a day for 2 days (dogs) or 10 mg per kg daily for 10 days (cats) is effective.

- Control is impractical without indoor confinement of animals.

Protozoa
Circulatory System

BABESIA AND THEILERIA SPP.

- Numerous species worldwide; species important to North America include *Babesia canis* (dogs), *B. bigemina* (cattle), *B. caballi*, and *Theileria equi* (horses).

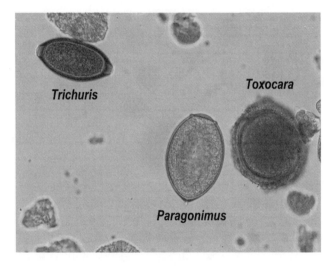

Figure 7–1 Fecal flotation from a dog with *P. kellicotti, T. canis,* and *T. vulpis* (200×).

Life Cycle

- Indirect.
- Definitive host: ixodid ticks.
- *Babesia*: all stages of ticks can transmit the organism; ticks become infected when ingesting a blood meal; gamonts fuse to form motile zygotes that invade various tissues; those invading oocytes result in transovarial transmission to the next tick generation; those invading salivary glands develop sporozoites that are passed to the mammalian host with the next blood meal; sporozoites penetrate erythrocytes, undergo asexual reproduction, and leave the cell to invade new cells; eventually, some organisms form gamonts, while others continue asexual reproduction; this cycle of reproduction and infection of new cells continues until the host controls the infection or dies; calves and colts are much less susceptible than older animals, but pups are more susceptible; prepatent period is 7–14 days.
- *Theileria*: life cycle as for *Babesia* except the motile zygotes only invade the salivary glands of the tick (no transovarian transmission occurs so larvae cannot transmit organisms) and sporozoites invade mammalian lymphocytes prior to infecting erythrocytes; prepatent period is 12–14 days.

Pathogenesis and Clinical Signs

- *Babesia* spp.: massive destruction of erythrocytes occurs during parasite development; infections are characterized by fever, anemia, and icterus; other clinical signs include hemoglobinemia, hemoglobinuria (except *B. caballi*), splenomegaly.

- *Theileria equi*: massive destruction of erythrocytes occurs during parasite development; clinical signs may include fever, depression, inappetence, anemia, icterus, hemoglobinuria, death.

Diagnosis

ANTEMORTEM

- *Babesia* spp.: may find erythrocytes with two or multiples of two organisms on blood films stained with Romanowsky stains (e.g., Giemsa); after acute phase, specialized serologic tests are needed. Note: *Babesia bigemina* has been eradicated from the United States.
- *Theileria equi*: may find erythrocytes with four organisms in the shape of a Maltese cross on blood films stained with Romanowsky stains (e.g., Giemsa); after acute phase, specialized serologic tests are needed.

Treatment and Control

- Dogs: no drugs are available for routine clinical use in the United States.
- Horses: no drugs are approved for this in the United States.
- Control is best achieved through controlling tick infestations.

CYTAUXZOON FELIS

- Distributed in the south-central United States in felids; sporadic occurrence, but uniformly fatal to domestic cats.

Life Cycle

- Indirect.
- Intermediate host: *Dermacentor variabilis* (experimental).
- Ticks acquiring infection as nymphs transmit the organism as adults (transstadial transmission); in ticks, development similar to that of *Theileria*; sporozoites transmitted via tick bite to definitive host, invade mononuclear cells lining venules of lungs, liver, spleen; grow into large meronts; merozoites eventually penetrate red blood cells.

Pathogenesis and Clinical Signs

- Infection of the mononuclear cells associated with the epithelia may result in partial or complete obstruction of small and medium veins in the lungs, spleen, and lymph nodes.
- Clinical signs include lethargy, depression, icterus, fever followed by hypothermia in the end stages of the disease; lymphadenopathy and splenomegaly are uncommon; death occurs in 1–4 days after onset of clinical signs in domestic cats.

Diagnosis

ANTEMORTEM AND POSTMORTEM

- May find erythrocytes containing organisms or mononuclear cells with meronts on stained blood smear.
- May find meronts in macrophages in stained impression smears of fine-needle aspirates of lymph node.

Treatment and Control

- No effective treatment currently exists; enrofloxacin for 10 days followed by tetracycline for 5 days was used in one cat that apparently survived infection.
- Control is best achieved by limiting tick infestations.

HEPATOZOON AMERICANUM

- Current known distribution is southeastern United States in domestic dogs and coyotes; prevalence unknown; moderate significance.

Life Cycle

- Indirect.
- Definitive host: *Amblyomma maculatum*, possibly *Rhipicephalus sanguineus*.
- Ticks acquire infection by ingesting organisms, presumably in leukocytes, with blood meal; oocysts form in the hemocoel.
- Dogs acquire infection by ingestion of infected ticks; asexual reproduction occurs within muscles; further details currently unknown.

Pathogenesis and Clinical Signs

- Tissue stages occur predominantly in skeletal and cardiac muscle; intense inflammatory response accompanies infection.
- Clinical signs include muscle pain resulting in gait abnormalities, depression, muscle atrophy, weakness, reluctance to rise, periosteal proliferation, and mucopurulent ocular discharge.

Diagnosis

ANTEMORTEM

- Demonstration of organism on muscle biopsy.
- Possibly demonstrate gamonts in circulating leukocytes with stained blood smear.

POSTMORTEM

- Demonstration of organism on tissue section.

Treatment and Control

- Most treatment protocols tried have some success in clearing the parasitemia and remission of clinical signs; however, most treatment regimens have not prevented relapses that tend to occur 3–6 months after treatment.
- Control is best achieved by limiting tick infestations.

8

Parasites of Other Organs

Nematodes

Eyes and Adnexa

THELAZIA SPP.

- Includes *Thelazia lacrymalis* in horses, *T. skrjabini,* and *T. gulosa* in cattle, and *T. californiensis* in dogs, cats, sheep, and humans.

- *Thelazia californiensis* found in North America; others have fairly cosmopolitan distribution; low significance.

Life Cycle

- Indirect.

- Intermediate host: muscoid flies, including the face fly *Musca autumnalis.*
- Adult females lay L_1; muscoid flies ingest larvae that develop to infective L_3 in approximately 2 weeks; infective L_3 transferred to definitive host when fly feeds again.
- Prepatent period is 10 days to 2 months.

Pathogenesis and Clinical Signs

- Generally nonpathogenic.
- Large numbers of worms may cause conjunctivitis; infections may also be predisposing factor for bacterial infections causing infectious keratoconjunctivitis; clinical signs of nematode infection include lacrimation, photophobia, and opaque cornea.

Diagnosis

ANTEMORTEM AND POSTMORTEM

- Adults are yellowish-white, slender, 1–2 cm in length; found in conjunctival sac, lacrimal ducts.

Treatment and Control

- Cattle: see Table 4–3.
- Dogs: ivermectin, SQ, at 0.2 mg per kg, has been effective.
- Control best achieved by proper fly control.

Skin, Subcutaneous and Connective Tissue

ACANTHOCHEILONEMA RECONDITUM

- Distributed in areas of Europe, Africa, and North America in canids; low significance except for need to differentiate from microfilariae of *D. immitis*.

Life Cycle

- Indirect.
- Intermediate host: fleas (*Ctenocephalids felis, C. canis, Pulex irritans*); also, ticks (*Rhipicephalus sanguineus*) and lice (*Heterodoxus spiniger*).
- Adults produce microfilariae (mff) that circulate in peripheral blood; flea ingests mff with blood meal; infective L_3 develops in 1–2 weeks and is passed to definitive host with next blood meal.
- Prepatent period is 2–3 months.

Pathogenesis and Clinical Signs

- Generally nonpathogenic.

Diagnosis

ANTEMORTEM

- Mff may be found on wet mount of blood or on stained, direct smear; Knott's technique or commercial filter kits may be used to concentrate mff (preferred); must be differentiated from *D. immitis* (see Table 7–1).

POSTMORTEM
- Adults are very small and generally missed at necropsy.

Treatment and Control
- Generally do not treat dogs for infection.
- Flea control will reduce the prevalence of this parasite.

STEPHANOFILARIA STILESI
- Distribution includes cattle in North America; low significance.

Life Cycle
- Indirect.
- Intermediate host: horn fly (*Haematobia irritans*).
- Adults live in dermis of midventral abdomen; produce mff that are ingested as flies feed; infective L_3 develops in 18–21 days; definitive host infected when the fly feeds again.
- Prepatent period is 6–8 weeks.

Pathogenesis and Clinical Signs
- Causes circumscribed dermatitis that begins in calves 8–10 months old and lasts for years; lesions start as small papules that coalesce to form larger lesions that are moist and/or hemorrhagic; as lesions resolve, the skin becomes thickened, dry, and hairless; eventually, the skin regains normal texture but remains hairless.

- Open lesions are usually present in cattle <3 years of age.
- Economic loss from condemnation of hides.

Diagnosis
ANTEMORTEM AND POSTMORTEM
- Usually based on typical lesions on ventral midline between navel and brisket; can find mff in a deep skin scrape or mff and adults in biopsy or tissue sections.

Treatment and Control
- Generally do not treat cattle for infection.
- Fly control is more important in preventing transmission.

ONCHOCERCA SPP.
- Includes *Onchocerca cervicalis* in horses and donkeys, and *O. gutturosa* and *O. lienalis* in cattle.
- Worldwide distribution; low significance.

Life Cycle
- Indirect.
- Intermediate hosts: blackflies (*Simulium* spp.) for *O. gutturosa* and *O. lienalis*; biting midges (*Culicoides* spp.) for *O. cervicalis*.
- Intermediate host ingests mff; develops to infective L_3 in 2–3 weeks; definitive host infected when infected arthropod feeds again; larvae migrate to final sites and develop to adults.

- Prepatent period is approximately 16 months for *O. cervicalis.*

Pathogenesis and Clinical Signs

- Adults are nonpathogenic as are mff in cattle.
- In horses, dying mff release antigens resulting in a hypersensitivity reaction; clinical signs may include alopecia, erythema, crusting with or without pruritis; must be differentiated from hypersensitivity reaction to biting flies.
- Aberrant infections in or near the eye of dogs have been reported; a few zoonotic cases have been reported in humans in North America.

Diagnosis

ANTEMORTEM

- Full-thickness skin biopsy soaked in warm saline for 6–12 hours; larvae leave samples and can be found in the sediment.
- Mff are found in the dermis of the ventral thorax and abdomen as well as head, neck, withers, and eye (*O. cervicalis*), the neck and back (*O. gutturosa*), or the ventral midline, especially near the umbilicus (*O. lienalis*).

POSTMORTEM

- Adults are slender, white, up to 5.5 cm in length; found in the ligamentum nuchae (*O. cervicalis, O. gutturosa*) or gastrosplenic ligament (*O. lienalis*).

Treatment and Control

- Generally do not treat domestic animals for infection.

- A single SQ injection of ivermectin at 0.2 mg per kg was effective in controlling dermatitis by killing mff in horses; post-treatment reactions to dying mff may occur; moxidectin at 0.3–0.5 mg per kg will eliminate mff from the blood of infected horses.

DRACUNCULUS INSIGNIS

- Distributed in North America in raccoons, mink, dogs, and cats; low significance.

Life Cycle

- Indirect.

- Intermediate host: copepod.

- Paratenic host: tadpoles/frogs.

- First-stage larvae are released into the water and ingested by the copepod; develop to infective L_3 in 13–16 days.

- Definitive host acquires infection by drinking water containing infected copepods or ingesting paratenic host (may be the most common route); larvae penetrate the small intestine and migrate to the subcutaneous tissues of the thorax, abdomen, and inguinal area; molt and mature in approximately 65 days; males die soon after mating; females may migrate to the subcutanous tissues of the limbs; nodules form that ulcerate at the location of the anterior end of the worm; whenever ulcer contacts water, the worm projects out of the ulcer, prolapses the uterus, and releases larvae into the water.

- Prepatent period approximately 200 days.

Pathogenesis and Clinical Signs

- Clinical signs include pruritic, painful, chronic nodules or abscesses, especially on the limbs or abdomen with or without ulceration; urticaria and fever may also occur.

Diagnosis

ANTEMORTEM AND POSTMORTEM

- May find L_1 in impression smears of discharge from lesions; larvae are 500–760 μm in length, with esophagus, intestinal tract, and anus, with distinctly prominent long, pointed tails; characteristics allow differentiation from mff.

- Can remove adults from nodules; females are up to 120 cm in length; presence of characteristic larvae in utero will allow differentiation from other subcutaneous nematodes.

Treatment and Control

- Treatment consists of removal of the worm; chemotherapy is ineffective.

- Prevent predation and scavenging whenever possible.

Peritoneum and Peritoneal Cavity

SETARIA SPP.

- Includes *S. equina* in equids and *S. labiatopapillosa* in ruminants.
- Cosmopolitan distribution; low significance.
- Common name: abdominal worm.

Life Cycle

- Indirect.
- Intermediate host: mosquitoes.
- Adults of both species live in the peritoneal cavity of their hosts; mff are found in the blood and ingested by mosquitoes during a blood meal; become infective L_3 in 10–15 days; transmitted to definitive host with next blood meal.
- Prepatent period is 8–10 months.

Pathogenesis and Clinical Signs

- Adults are nonpathogenic although can be associated with a fibrinous peritonitis.
- Migrating larval *S. labiatopapillosa* may reach ectopic sites such as brain and spinal cord causing encephalomyelomalacia of sheep and horses (not reported in the United States).

Diagnosis

ANTEMORTEM
- Can find mff using same techniques as for *A. reconditum*.
- Occasionally, adults may be obtained during peritoneal tap or found during abdominal surgery.

POSTMORTEM
- Worms are white, long, slender, 4–13 cm; found free in abdominal cavity, occasionally thoracic cavity (*S. equina*).

Treatment and Control

- Generally do not treat domestic animals for infection.

Musculoskeletal System

TRICHINELLA SPIRALIS
- Worldwide distribution in a variety of mammals including pigs and humans; moderate significance to veterinary medicine but may be highly significant to public health.

Life Cycle

- Direct.
- Unique in that the adult and infective larvae occur within the same host with no intervening free-living stage.
- Adults live in the small intestine; females lay larvae that penetrate the wall of the intestine and enter venules and

lymphatics; migrates via the circulatory system to skeletal muscles; preferred sites are diaphragmatic, intercostal, masseter, and tongue muscles; larvae enter myocytes, coil and grow, but do not molt; becomes infective L_1 in approximately 15 days.

- Definitive host acquires infection by eating infected muscle tissue; larvae penetrate into the small intestinal mucosa, molt, and mature 36–40 hours postinfection; larviposition begins 5–6 days postinfection; adult infections are short-lived (4–6 weeks) and self-terminating.

- Sylvatic cycle involves wild carnivorous or omnivorous mammals and their prey species; domestic cycle occurs when prey species, such as rats, are ingested by pigs, dogs, or cats; human infections occur by ingesting undercooked or raw meat such as pork, pork products, horse, or bear meat.

Pathogenesis and Clinical Signs

- Larvae in the myocyte become encapsulated by a host-derived membrane in approximately 3 months; cysts may calcify as they age but some larvae will remain alive for 2 or more years.

- Infections of domestic animals are generally inapparent; may be misdiagnosed.

- Infections in humans may be inapparent or fatal; symptoms may include abdominal pain, diarrhea, nausea, fever, myalgia, and malaise.

Diagnosis

ANTEMORTEM

- Difficult; commercial enzyme immunoassays for use with serum, whole blood, or tissue fluids are available in the United States for testing pigs.

POSTMORTEM

- Several samples of diaphragm (total of 1–5 gm) are pressed between glass slides and examined at approximately 40× for larvae; detects approximately 3 larvae per gram of muscle.

- Artificial digestion fluid can be used to break down muscle tissue to free larvae that can be seen in sediment with light microscopy.

Treatment and Control

- Generally do not treat domestic animals for infection.

- Control on-farm requires good hygiene; heat-treat (at least 60°C for 60 min) scraps fed to pigs; a new system of food safety to certify pigs as free of the parasite on-farm is being implemented in the United States.

- For humans, the best control is proper cooking of meat; larvae die around 57°C, so cooking of meat to an internal temperature of 77°C is recommended; freezing also kills larvae, but cuts must be ≤15 cm thick and frozen at −15°C for at least 20 days (freezing does not kill some of the other species of *Trichinella* such as *T. nativa*).

Urogenital System

STEPHANURUS DENTATUS

- Distributed in domestic and wild pigs in tropical and subtropical regions; locally significant in pigs raised in outdoor situations.

- Common name: kidney worm.

Life Cycle

- Direct; indirect with paratenic host.

- Eggs passed in urine; L_1 develops and hatches; infective L_3 develops in approximately 4 days; paratenic host becomes infected by ingesting infective L_3.

- Pig acquires infection through either the percutaneous route, ingestion of infective L_3 directly or in paratenic host, or transplacental transmission; ingested larvae penetrate the stomach wall, molt to L_4, and migrate to liver via portal circulation; percutaneous larvae molt to L_4 in skin and migrate to liver via the lungs and systemic circulation; larvae migrate in the liver for 3–9 months, molt, and penetrate the liver capsule to migrate to the perirenal tissues and wall of the ureters where they mature.

- Prepatent period is 9–16 months; may live 3 or more years.

Pathogenesis and Clinical Signs

- Migrating larvae are more pathogenic than adults with the liver most severely affected; hypertrophy, cirrhosis, and thrombosis of hepatic vessels may occur; larvae may also migrate to ectopic sites where they are encapsulated.

- Adults are enclosed in fibrous cysts connected by channels to ureters or renal pelvis; adults may cause peritonitis, urethritis, and cystitis.

- Clinical signs may include inappetence, decreased weight gain or weight loss, emaciation, ascites; death is rare.

Diagnosis

ANTEMORTEM

- Can find trichostrongyle-type eggs in urine sediment.

- Eggs are ellipsoidal, broad, thin-shelled, 90–120 × 43–70 μm, containing morula with 32–64 cells.

POSTMORTEM

- Adults are pinkish, stout, 2–4.5 cm in length; found in capsules in perirenal fat, ureter walls, and adjacent tissues.

Treatment and Control

- See Table 4–1 for treatment.

- Because of the long prepatent period, can run gilts through a single breeding cycle before egg shedding begins; this progressively eradicates the source of infection.

DIOCTOPHYMA RENALE

- Distributed in southern Europe, North and South

America in mink, marten, polecat, weasels, canids, cats; occasionally reported in cattle, pigs, and humans.

- Common name: giant kidney worm.

Life Cycle

- Indirect.
- Intermediate host: aquatic oligochaete.
- Paratenic host: frogs and fish (e.g., bullhead, pike).
- Eggs are passed in the urine; L_1 develops within the egg in approximately 1 month; oligochaete ingests egg containing L_1; develops to infective L_3 in 2–4 months.
- Definitive host becomes infected by ingesting infected oligochaete or, more likely, through ingestion of paratenic host; larvae penetrate stomach wall, migrate through the liver and body cavity to the kidney, molt, and mature to adults.
- Prepatent period: 3.5–6 months.

Pathogenesis and Clinical Signs

- Larval migration through the stomach cause hemorrhages, inflammation, and fibrosis; migration through the liver causes necrotic tracks that fibrose; if females remain in the abdominal cavity, they may release large numbers of unfertilized eggs causing peritonitis; infection of the kidney causes atrophy and fibrosis; hydronephrosis may or may not occur.

- Infection may be inapparent; clinical signs may include abdominal and lumbar pain, inappetence, vomiting, hematuria, uremia, and polydipsia.

Diagnosis

ANTEMORTEM

- Eggs may be found in urine sediment.
- Eggs are barrel-shaped, with thick, yellow-brown, pitted shell except at poles that are clear ("bipolar plugs"), $71–84 \times 46–52$ μm.

POSTMORTEM

- Worms are red, very large—females are up to 1 m in length and 1 cm in width; found in the abdominal cavity or kidney.

Treatment and Control

- Treatment consists of surgical removal of the parasite and affected kidney, if necessary.
- Prevent predation and scavenging whenever possible.

PEARSONEMA PLICA; P. FELISCATI

- Probably worldwide in distribution in a variety of carnivores and omnivores; low significance.

Life Cycle

- Indirect; known for *P. plica* only.

- Eggs are passed in the feces; infective L_1 develops in approximately 2 weeks and hatches after ingestion by earthworms; larval development beyond L_1 does not occur.

- Definitive host acquires infection by ingesting infected earthworms.

- Prepatent period is approximately 2 months.

Pathogenesis and Clinical Signs

- Generally not pathogenic.

Diagnosis

ANTEMORTEM

- Eggs may be found in urine sediment or on fecal flotation of urine-contaminated feces.

- Eggs are typical capillarid type, clear to yellow, approximately 65×25 µm, with flattened bipolar plugs on each end.

POSTMORTEM

- Adults live in the urinary bladder; adult worms are hair-like and are generally missed during gross necropsy; rather, they may be found on histologic sections.

Treatment and Control

- Fenbendazole at 50 mg per kg daily for 3 days and ivermectin at 0.2 mg per kg once have been successful in dogs.

Cestodes

Musculoskeletal System

TAENIA SPP.

- Includes *Taenia saginata* (beef tapeworm) and *T. solium* (pork tapeworm) of humans; low to moderate significance to veterinary medicine, but highly significant to public health.

- Worldwide distribution although *T. solium* has become rare in Europe and North America.

Life Cycle

- Indirect.

- Intermediate host: cattle (*T. saginata*); domestic and wild swine, humans, occasionally dogs (*T. solium*).

- Metacestode: cysticercus.

- *Taenia saginata*: gravid proglottids are passed in feces or migrate out of the anus; eggs are shed from proglottid; cattle become infected by ingesting eggs when feeding; oncospheres leave eggs, penetrate intestinal wall, and travel to cardiac and skeletal muscles via the circulatory system; cysticerci develop and become infective in 8–16 weeks; live up to 2 years; dead cysticerci may calcify; occasionally, may find cysticerci in brain, lungs, liver, and other sites; humans acquire infection by ingesting undercooked or raw beef; scavenging birds may disseminate eggs.

- *Taenia solium*: similar to *T. saginata*; cysticerci may be found in striated muscle, heart, liver, lung, kidney, subcutaneous tissues, CNS; become infective in 10–12 weeks; may survive lifelong in the pig; humans are definitive host but can also become infected with cysticerci by release of eggs from gravid proglottids transferred to the stomach from the duodenum by reverse peristalsis or by ingestion of eggs; neurocysticercosis or ocular cysticercosis may result.

Pathogenesis and Clinical Signs

- Infection with both adult and metacestode stages is usually inapparent.

- In dogs, infections with cysticerci of *T. solium* may result in neurologic disorders and death as a result of localizing in the brain.

- In humans, infections with cysticerci of *T. solium* may interfere with vision or cause neurologic disorders and death.

Diagnosis

ANTEMORTEM

- Can differentiate gravid proglottids of *T. solium* from those of *T. saginata*; however, it is unlikely the practitioner would be asked to do so.

- Serodiagnostic tests have been developed for pre-slaughter diagnosis of infections in pigs in countries outside the United States.

POSTMORTEM

- Cysticercus of *T. saginata* is white, ovoid, fluid-filled, up to 1 cm in diameter; invaginated scolex does not have a rostellum or hooks; dead, calcifying cysticerci are difficult to identify.

- Cysticercus of *T. solium* is white, ovoid, fluid-filled, up to 1.8 cm in diameter; invaginated scolex has a rostellum and hooks; dead cysticerci can be recognized by the presence of hooks.

Treatment and Control

- Treatment of domestic animals for larval cestodes is generally not attempted.

- Control methods include proper hygiene to prevent contamination of feed and water with human feces.

Trematodes

Liver

FASCIOLA HEPATICA

- Worldwide distribution in ruminants, pigs, and horses; occasionally in humans; distribution in North America centers on the Gulf Coast/southeastern states, Pacific Northwest (including Montana), and eastern Canada; highly significant to veterinary medicine; low significance to public health.

- Common name: liver fluke.

Life Cycle

- Indirect.

- Intermediate host: lymnaeid snails; require neutral, poorly drained soil.

- Eggs are passed with bile to intestine and out with the feces; miracidia develop in 10–12 days; require water to hatch; penetrate snail, undergo asexual development and produce cercariae in 1–2 months; one miracidium into a snail equals several hundred cercariae out of snail; leave and attach to vegetation where encyst becoming metacercariae; cercariae may also overwinter in snail.

- Definitive host acquires infection by ingesting metacercariae on vegetation; fluke penetrates the small intestine to abdominal cavity, migrates to and penetrates liver in 4–6 days; migrates throughout liver for 4–7 weeks and then enters bile ducts and matures.

- Prepatent period is 8–12 weeks; may live for several years.

- In temperate regions, carrier animals important in contaminating pastures in the spring; metacercariae appear during late summer into fall.

- In mild regions, infected snails may overwinter; metacercariae may appear during spring to early summer; spring occurrence depends on moisture and snail activity the preceding fall; carrier animals also important in maintaining pasture contamination.

Pathogenesis and Clinical Signs

- Migration of immature flukes causes traumatic hepatitis and hemorrhage; anemia may result; migratory tracts eventually heal by fibrosis.

- Adults ingest blood and may also cause anemia; presence of adults causes extensive proliferation of the bile duct epithelium, cholangitis, and necrosis of the ductal wall; fibrosis of the lamina propria of the bile duct occurs that may eventually calcify.

- Clinical disease occurs in four forms:

  1. *Acute*—caused by short-term intake of massive numbers of metacercariae that invade the liver all at once; clinical signs include inappetence, weight loss, abdominal pain, anemia, ascites, depression, sudden death; course is only a few days; occurs primarily in sheep and goats.

  2. *Subacute*—also caused by intake of massive numbers of metacercariae, but over a longer period of time; clinical signs include inappetence, decreased weight gain or weight loss, progressive hemorrhagic anemia, liver failure, and death; course is 4–8 weeks.

  3. *Chronic*—caused by intake of moderate numbers of metacercariae over an extended period of time; clinical signs include decreased feed intake and weight gain, reduced milk yield, anemia, emaciation, submandibular edema, ascites; cattle tend to exhibit chronic disease.

4. *Subclinical*—caused by intake of low numbers of metacercariae over a long period of time; moderate cholangitis occurs without apparent clinical signs.

Diagnosis

ANTEMORTEM

- May find eggs on fecal sedimentation during chronic and subclinical infections, possibly subacute infections also.
- Eggs are oval, operculate, yellow, $130–150 \times 65–90$ µm.

POSTMORTEM

- Mature flukes may be found within the bile ducts; flukes are leaf-shaped, greenish-brown, $2–4 \times 1–1.5$ cm; with conical anterior end and shoulders.
- Immature flukes (up to 7 mm in length) may be difficult to find within the liver parenchyma; requires sequential slicing of the liver and expressing flukes from cut surfaces.

Treatment and Control

- See Table 4–3 for treatment of cattle; albendazole at 7.5 mg per kg in sheep and 15 mg per kg in goats has been used.
- Strategic use of anthelmintics is cornerstone of control programs; purpose is to remove parasites before animal productivity is affected and to prevent egg shedding that subsequently contaminates pastures; the timing, frequency, and choice of anthelmintic

vary based on the transmission patterns in each geographic region.

- Grazing management should avoid high-risk areas during periods of transmission; may need to fence off areas of snail habitat; control of snails themselves through draining of habitat or use of molluscicides is impractical in most cases.

FASCIOLOIDES MAGNA

- Distributed in North America, central Europe, Mexico, and South Africa; cervids are the usual definitive hosts; cattle, sheep, and goats may be accidentally infected; low to moderate significance.
- Common name: large American liver fluke.

Life Cycle

- Indirect.
- Intermediate host: freshwater lymnaeid snails.
- In cervid definitive host, life cycle is essentially as for *F. hepatica.*
- Prepatent period is approximately 8 months.
- Patency is generally not achieved in cattle or sheep (see Pathogenesis and Clinical Signs).

Pathogenesis and Clinical Signs

- Cervids: infections are inapparent; flukes are encapsulated by a thin-walled cyst with channels to the bile ducts; eggs leave the cysts via these channels.

- Cattle: infections tend to be inapparent; flukes reach the liver and are encapsulated in cysts that usually do not communicate with the bile ducts; eggs generally are not passed out of cysts.

- Sheep, goats: flukes tend to migrate continuously within the liver as well as to ectopic sites such as the lungs; traumatic hepatitis results, which is fatal before flukes mature.

Diagnosis

ANTEMORTEM
- May find eggs on fecal sedimentation of deer feces; eggs are oval, operculate, yellow, 110–160 × ~ 75 μm.

POSTMORTEM
- Mature flukes may be found in cysts in liver of cervids and cattle or within the liver parenchyma or other organs of sheep and goats; flukes are leaf-shaped with no demarcated anterior cone, thick, up to 10 cm in length by 2.5 cm in width.

Treatment and Control

- Clorsulon at 20 mg per kg in both sheep and cattle has been used.

- Prevention is best achieved by not grazing sheep in endemic areas; avoid grazing cattle in high-risk areas during transmission.

DICROCOELIUM DENDRITICUM

- Worldwide distribution, except Australia, in cattle, sheep, and goats; sporadic occurrence, moderate significance.

Life Cycle

- Indirect.

- First intermediate host: terrestrial snails.

- Second intermediate host: ants.

- Embryonated eggs are passed with the feces and ingested by snails; cercariae develop in 3–4 months, are shed by the snail, and clump together in slime-balls; ants eat slime-balls and metacercariae form in 26–62 days; most develop in the hemocoel, but some lodge in the subesophageal ganglion; this causes tetanic spasms of the mouthparts as temperatures decrease, which locks the ant onto herbage overnight; ants are then available to grazing animals the following morning.

- Definitive host acquires infection by ingesting ant containing metacercariae; flukes enter the liver by migrating up the bile ducts from the small intestine.

- Prepatent period is 47–54 days; may live for 6 years or longer.

Pathogenesis and Clinical Signs

- Pathologic changes increase in severity as infection increases in age; advanced infections can cause hepatic cirrhosis and proliferation of bile duct epithelium.

- Clinical signs in young animals are usually not present; in sheep, may cause anemia, edema, decreased wool production, and lactation.

Diagnosis

ANTEMORTEM
- Eggs may be found on fecal sedimentation.
- Eggs are brown, operculated, oval, 36–46 × 10–20 μm, containing miracidia; operculum may be difficult to see.

POSTMORTEM
- The flukes are flattened, leaf-like, 6–10 × 1.5–2.5 mm; found in bile ducts; because of their small size, they may be missed at necropsy.

Treatment and Control

- Generally do not treat domestic animals for infection; if heavy infections are present, can use albendazole at 15–20 mg per kg once or 7.5 mg per kg once and repeated 2–3 weeks later; fenbendazole at 100–150 mg per kg has also been used.

PLATYNOSOMUM FASTOSUM
- Distributed in southern North America through Central and South America, West Africa, Malaysia, and Pacific Islands in cats; usually low significance except in highly endemic areas.

Life Cycle

- Indirect.
- First intermediate host: terrestrial snails.
- Second intermediate host: sowbugs, woodlice, lizards.
- Paratenic host: lizards, frogs.
- Embryonated eggs are passed with the feces and ingested by snails; sporocysts containing cercariae are shed by snail and ingested by second intermediate host in which metacercariae form.
- Cats acquire infection by ingesting infected lizards (hence the name "lizard poisoning disease"); flukes migrate from the small intestine up the common bile duct.
- Prepatent period is 2–3 months.

Pathogenesis and Clinical Signs

- Infections are usually inapparent with only a short-term inappetence occurring.
- Heavy infections can cause proliferative cholangitis and cirrhosis.
- Clinical signs may include anorexia, icterus, enlarged liver, diarrhea, vomiting, and death.

Diagnosis

ANTEMORTEM

- Eggs may be found on fecal sedimentation; fecal flotation may be ineffective.

- Eggs are brown, operculated, oval, 35–50 × 20–35 μm, containing miracidia.

POSTMORTEM
- Adults live in bile ducts, gallbladder, and pancreas; worms are very small and generally not seen at necropsy; rather, may find them on histologic section.

Treatment and Control
- Praziquantel at 20 mg per kg has been used.
- Prevent predation and scavenging whenever possible.

Protozoa
Urogenital System
TRITRICHOMONAS FOETUS
- Worldwide distribution in cattle; moderate significance.

Life Cycle
- Direct.
- Transmitted by coitus; in cows, parasites first multiply in secretions of the vagina (2 weeks), then the uterus; in bulls, parasites colonize the secretions of the epithelial lining of the penis, prepuce, and distal urethra; prevalence increases in bulls >4 years old.

Pathogenesis and Clinical Signs
- Bulls: infection is inapparent; remains infected for life.

- Cows: causes vaginitis and endometritis; clinical signs include early embryonic death, abortion, pyometra, fetal maceration, or infertility; infection is self-limiting with clearance occurring within 20 weeks of primary infection and 10 weeks of secondary infection.

Diagnosis
ANTEMORTEM AND POSTMORTEM
- Examination of wet mounts and/or stained smears of bull smegma, vaginal secretions or washings, or aborted material for organisms; may want to culture material to increase numbers; because nonpathogenic trichomonads live in the intestinal tract, must be careful not to contaminate sample with feces.

- Organisms are pear-shaped, 10–25 × 3–15 μm, with three anterior flagella, undulating membrane, and trailing posterior flagellum.

- A single positive test is adequate to diagnose herd infections but three or more negative tests are necessary to ensure individual bulls are not infected.

Treatment and Control
- Generally do not treat cattle for infection.
- Control measures: replace older bulls with younger bulls; do not borrow or lease bulls; culture all newly purchased bulls regardless of age and bulls 2 weeks after the breeding season—cull those that are positive; use artificial

insemination whenever possible using semen from a facility that tests for the parasite; vaccinate cows and heifers if the threat of exposure is unavoidable.

Liver

HISTOMONAS MELEAGRIDIS

- Worldwide distribution in gallinaceous birds; locally significant in free-ranging birds.

- Common name: blackhead.

Life Cycle

- Direct; indirect with *Heterakis gallinarum* or earthworm paratenic host.

- Trophozoites are passed in the feces or in the eggs of *H. gallinarum* (nematodes ingest trophozoites that infect oocytes); primary means of transmission is ingestion of trophozoites in eggs of *H. gallinarum* or in eggs of *H. gallinarum* in earthworms; trophozoites die quickly (within hours) but it is possible they can be ingested with contaminated food or water.

- Remains in flagellated form in cecal lumen approximately 1 week; penetrates subepithelial tissues appearing as a round form without flagellum; carried via circulation to liver 10–12 days postinfection.

Pathogenesis and Clinical Signs

- Chickens: nonpathogenic.

- Turkeys: causes inflammation and ulcers in the ceca; cores of necrotic tissue, exudate, and parasites plug ceca; in liver, causes characteristic circular, yellow-green areas of necrosis with a depressed center; clinical signs include depression, inappetence, sulfur-colored droppings, cyanosis of the head (hence the common name), death.

Diagnosis

ANTEMORTEM
- None.

POSTMORTEM
- Examination of fresh or fixed impression smears obtained from the edge of cecal or liver lesions for organisms; may also be able to find organisms in histological sections.

Treatment and Control

- Modern, intensive management has decreased the incidence of this parasite; separate turkeys from chickens and poults from adults; avoid contaminated ground and adhere to strict sanitation; reuse of litter may lead to build-up of *H. meleagridis* eggs; treat chickens for *H. meleagridis*.

Nervous System

SARCOCYSTIS NEURONA

- Distribution limited to Canada, North, Central and South America; high significance to equine industry.

Life Cycle

- Indirect.
- Intermediate host: unknown.
- Definitive host are opossums; horses presumed to acquire infection by ingesting infective sporocysts; parasite localizes in CNS; parasite apparently does not develop to the infective stage in equids and they are considered dead-end hosts.
- Overall, seroprevalence is approximately 50%, but can be as high as 80% in older animals; true incidence of clinical disease is unknown, but much lower than seroprevalence.

Pathogenesis and Clinical Signs

- Causes a necrotizing encephalomyelitis; affects both white and gray matter.
- Clinical signs vary depending on the location of the organisms; may include ataxia, paresis, rapid muscle atrophy, head tilt, muzzle deviation, dysphagia.

Diagnosis

ANTEMORTEM
- No single definitive diagnostic test exists; Western blot assay for *S. neurona* antibody in CSF indicates exposure.

POSTMORTEM
- Difficult; gross lesions (yellowish or red swollen areas) in neural tissue may or may not be present; may or may not be able to identify organism in histologic sections.

Treatment and Control

- Treatment may or may not be effective; for treatment protocol, consult the current literature.
- Prevention is based on eliminating sporocyst contamination of feed and water.

Glossary

Aberrant Host: Host in which parasite can develop, but the timing is prolonged or the numbers that establish are low.

Aberrant Parasite: Parasite that wanders from its usual site of infection into an unusual organ or location in its normal definitive host.

Abnormal Host: Host in which the parasite does not fully develop (e.g., *Sarcocystis neurona* in horses).

Acariasis: Infestation with ticks or mites.

Arrested Development: Temporary cessation of larval development occurring in nematodes; may occur at the L_3 stage (e.g., *Ancylostoma*), the early L_4 stage (e.g., *Ostertagia*, small strongyles), or the immature adult stage (e.g., *Dictyocaulus*).

Bot Fly: Refers to adults of the grub-like dipterous larvae that parasitize mammals.

Commensalism: Symbiotic relationship in which one member benefits and the other neither benefits nor is harmed.

Complex (Complete) Metamorphosis: In arthropods, developmental stages do not resemble the adult stage.

Definitive Host: Host in which the sexually mature parasite occurs.

Direct Life Cycle: Cycle in which no intermediate host is needed for transmission of the parasite from one definitive host to another.

Ectoparasite: Parasite that lives on the body of its host.

Endoparasite: Parasite that lives within the body of its host.

Facultative Parasite: Organisms that are normally nonparasitic (free-living), but can become parasitic in certain hosts or under certain circumstances.

Indirect Life Cycle: Cycle in which one or more intermediate or paratenic hosts are needed for transmission of the parasite from one definitive host to another.

Infective Stage: The developmental stage of a parasite that is capable of establishing in the definitive host.

Intermediate Host: Host in which preadult or asexually reproducing stages of the organism occur; intermediate hosts are *required* for the completion of the life cycle of the parasite (e.g., mosquitoes for *Dirofilaria immitis*).

Metacestode: Refers to the developmental stages of tapeworm within the intermediate host.

Mutualism: Symbiotic relationship in which both organisms benefit.

Myiasis: Infestation with fly larvae; may be obligatory (animal host is *required* for completion of the life cycle) or facultative (animal host is *not required* for completion of the life cycle).

Obligatory Parasite: Organisms that cannot lead a totally free-living existence.

Parasitism: Symbiotic relationship in which one member, the parasite, lives on or within the other member and derives nutritional benefit from the other member; the relationship is usually considered harmful to the other member.

Paratenic Host: Host in which the parasite stage or stages can live but in which little or no development occurs; host is *not required* in order for the parasite to complete its life cycle (e.g., mice for *Toxocara mystax*).

Pediculosis: Infestation with lice.

Phoresis: Symbiotic relationship in which one member is mechanically carried by the other member.

Prepatent Period: The time from acquisition of the infective stage of a parasite to detection of the diagnostic stage; varies with, among other things, the technique used to detect the diagnostic stage and numbers of reproductively active parasites.

Pseudoparasite: Objects that are present in feces that may be mistaken for parasitic stages.

Simple (Incomplete) Metamorphosis: In arthropods, developmental stages do resemble the adult stage.

Site: The tissue, organ, or part of the host where the parasite is normally found.

Species: An interbreeding population that is reproductively isolated from other such populations.

Symbiosis: Any association, either temporary or permanent, between two or more living organisms of different species.

Transovarial Transmission: Pathogen acquired by adult female ticks infects the ovaries and passes with the eggs to the larvae; important for one-host ticks.

Transstadial Transmission: Pathogen acquired by tick remains in it as it molts from one stage to the next; important for two- or three-host ticks.

Vector: Arthropod that transmits a pathogen from one host to another. Two types: (1) mechanical vector—transmits infective organism to recipient without development or multiplication of the organism; and (2) biological vector—infective organisms undergo development prior to transmission to the next host.

Warble: A subcutaneous swelling in which the larva of certain bot flies lives (e.g., *Hypoderma*).

Zoonosis: Any disease or parasite that is transmissible from animals to humans.

References and Suggested Reading

Anderson DL, Roberson EL. Gastrointestinal and respiratory parasitism in Georgia goats. *Agri-Practice* 1996;17:20–24.

Anderson RC. *Nematode Parasites of Vertebrates: Their Development and Transmission.* Wallingford, CT: CAB International; 1992.

Arrioja-Dechert A, ed. *Compendium of Veterinary Products.* 5th ed. Port Huron: North American Compendiums; 1999.

Atkinson R, Harper PAW, Reichel MP, Ellis JT. Progress in the serodiagnosis of *Neospora caninum* infections of cattle. *Parasitol Today* 2000;16:110–114.

Barger IA. Influence of sex and reproductive status on susceptibility of ruminants to nematode parasitism. *Int J Parasitol* 1993;23:463–469.

Barr SC, Jamrosz GF, Hornbuckle WE, Bowman DD, Fayer R. Use of paromomycin for treatment of cryptosporidiosis in a cat. *J Am Vet Med Assoc* 1994;205:1742–1743.

Barriga OO. *Veterinary Parasitology for Practitioners.* 2nd ed. Edina: Burgess Publishing, 1997.

Baudena MA, Chapman MR, French DD, Klei TR. Seasonal development and survival of equine cyathostome larvae on pasture in south Louisiana. *Vet Parasitol* 2000;88:51–60.

Bello TR, Abell JE. Are equine tapeworms an emerging disease? A retrospective study. *J Equine Vet Sci* 1999;19:723–727.

Bentz BG, Carter WG, Tobin T. Diagnosing equine protozoal myeloencephalitis: complicating factors. *Compen Contin Educ Pract Vet* 1999;21:975–981.

Beyer TA, Pinckney RD, Cooley AJ. Massive *Dracunculus insignis* infection in a dog. *J Am Vet Med Assoc* 1999;214:366–368.

Bowman DD. *Georgis' Parasitology for Veterinarians*. 7th ed. Philadelphia: W.B. Saunders; 1999.

Brawner Jr. WR, Dillon AR, Robertson-Plouch CK, Guerrero J. Radiographic diagnosis of feline heartworm disease and correlation to other clinical criteria: results of a multicenter clinical case study. *Vet Ther: Res Appl Vet Med* 2000;1:81–87.

Bredal WP. *Pneumonyssoides caninum* infection—a risk factor for gastric dilatation-volvulus in dogs. *Vet Res Commun* 1998;22:225–231.

Bredal W, Vollset I. Use of milbemycin oxime in the treatment of dogs with nasal mite (*Pneumonyssoides caninum*) infection. *J Small Anim Pract* 1998;39:126–130.

Burks BS. Parasitic pneumonitis in horses. *Compen Contin Educ Pract Vet* 1999;20:378–383.

Buxton D. Protozoan infections (*Toxoplasma gondii, Neospora caninum* and *Sarcocystis* spp.) in sheep and goats: recent advances. *Vet Res* 1998;29:289–310.

Campbell BG. *Trichuris* and other trichinelloid nematodes of dogs and cats in the United States. *Compen Contin Educ Pract Vet* 1991;13:769–778.

Chartier C, Mallereau M-P, Naciri M. Prophylaxis using paromomycin of natural cryptosporidial infection in neonatal kids. *Prevent Vet Med* 1996;25:357–361.

Chen C. A short-tailed demodectic mite and *Demodex canis* infestation in a Chihuahua dog. *Vet Dermatol* 1995;6:227–229.

Chesney CJ. Short form of *Demodex* species mite in the dog: occurrence and measurements. *J Small Anim Pract* 1999;40:58–61.

Clyde VS. Practical treatment and control of common ectoparasites in exotic pets. *Vet Med* 1996;91:632–637.

Clyde VS. Practical treatment and control of common endoparasites in exotic pets. *Vet Med* 1996;91:638–647.

Coles GC, Pearson GR. *Gasterophilus nasalis* infection: prevalence and pathological changes in equids in south-west England. *Vet Rec* 2000;146:222–223.

Coles GC, Brown SN, Trembath CM. Pyrantel-resistant large strongyles in racehorses. *Vet Rec* 1999;145:408.

Conboy G. Giardia. *Can Vet J* 1997;38:245–247.

Corwin RM, Nahm J. Veterinary Parasitology Website. 1997, last updated 1/10/00, URL:http:www.parasitology.org.

Craig TM. Coccidiosis in small ruminants. In: Weide KC, Weide KD, eds. *Small Ruminants for the Mixed Animal Practitioner.* Las Vegas: Western Veterinary Conference; 1998:41–45.

Craig TM. Ectoparasites of small ruminants. In: Weide KC, Weide KD, eds. *Small Ruminants for the Mixed Animal Practitioner.* Las Vegas: Western Veterinary Conference; 1998: 46–50.

Curtsinger DK, Carpenter JL, Turner JL. Gastritis caused by *Aonchotheca putorii* in a domestic cat. *J Am Vet Med Assoc* 1993;203:1153–1154.

Dangjin L. Study on a new egg count technique for *Macracanthorhynchus hirudinaceus* and *Ascaris suum. Vet Parasitol* 1996;61:113–117.

Deem SL. Infectious and parasitic diseases of raptors. *Compen Contin Educ Pract Vet* 1999;21:329–338.

Delucchi L, Castro E. Use of doramectin for treatment of notoedric mange in five cats. *J Am Vet Med Assoc* 2000;216: 215–216.

Denegri GM. Review of oribatid mites as intermediate hosts of tapeworms of the Anoplocephalidae. *Exp Appl Acarol* 1993; 17:567–580.

Desch Jr. CE, Stewart TB. *Demodex gatoi*: new species of hair follicle mite (Acari: Demodecidae) from the domestic cat (Carnivora: Felidae). *J Med Entomol* 1999;36:167–170.

Dillon R. Clinical significance of feline heartworm disease. *Vet Clin N Am: Small Anim Pract* 1998;28:1547–1564.

Divers TJ, Bowman DD, de LaHunta A. Equine protozoal myeloencephalitis: recent advances in diagnosis and treatment. *Vet CE Advisor, Suppl Vet Med* 2000:17.

Dryden MW. Biology of fleas of dogs and cats. *Compen Contin Educ Pract Vet* 1993;15:569–578.

Dubey JP. Intestinal protozoa infections. *Vet Clin N Am: Small Anim Pract* 1993;21:37–55.

Dubey JP. Advances in the life cycle of *Toxoplasma gondii*. *Int J Parasitol* 1998;28:1019–1024.

Dubey JP. Neosporosis in cattle: biology and economic impact. *J Am Vet Med Assoc* 1999;214:1160–1163.

Dubey JP. Recent advances in *Neospora* and neosporosis. *Vet Parasitol* 1999;84:349–367.

Dubey JP. Toxoplasmosis. In: Howard JL, Smith RA, eds. *Current Veterinary Therapy 4: Food Animal Practice*. Philadelphia: W.B. Saunders; 1999:431–433.

Dubey JP. Sarcocystosis. In: Howard JL, Smith RA, eds. *Current Veterinary Therapy 4: Food Animal Practice*. Philadelphia: W.B. Saunders; 1999:433–435.

Dubey JP, Lindsay DS. A review of *Neospora caninum* and neosporosis. *Vet Parasitol* 1996;67:1–59.

Dubey JP, Lindsay DS. Isolation in immunodeficient mice of *Sarcocystis neurona* from opossum (*Didelphis virginiana*) faeces, and its differentiation from *Sarcocystis falcatula*. *Int J Parasitol* 1998;28:1823–1828.

Eberhard ML, Brandt FH. The role of tadpoles and frogs as paratenic hosts in the life cycle of *Dracunculus insignis* (Nematoda: Dracunculoidea). *J Parasitol* 1995;81:792–793.

Eberhard ML, Ortega Y, Dial S, Schiller CA, Sears AW, Greiner E. Ocular *Onchocerca* infections in two dogs in western United States. *Vet Parasitol* 2000;90:333–338.

Engelbrecht NE, Yeatts RP, Slansky F. Palpebral myiasis causing preseptal cellulitis. *Arch Ophthalmol* 1998;116:684.

Eysker M. Dictyocaulosis in cattle. *Compen Contin Educ Pract Vet* 1994;16:669–675.

Fayer R, Ellis W. Paromomycin is effective as prophylaxis for cryptosporidiosis in dairy calves. *J Parasitol* 1993; 79:771–774.

Fayer R, Speer CA, Dubey JP. The general biology of *Cryptosporidium*. In: Fayer R, ed. *Cryptosporidium and Cryptosporidiosis*. Boca Raton, FL: CRC Press; 1997:1–41.

Fenger CK, Granstrom DE, Langemeier JL, Stamper S, Donahue JM, Patterson JL, Gajadhar AA, Marteniuk JV, Xiaomin A, Dubey JP. Identification of opossums (*Didelphis virginiana*) as the putative definitive host of *Sarcocystis neurona. J Parasitol* 1995;81:916–919.

Giovengo SL. Canine dracunculiasis. *Compen Contin Educ Pract Vet* 1993;15:726–729.

Goddard J. Human infestation with rodent botfly larvae: a new route of entry? *South Med J* 1997;90:254–255.

Goodwin J-K. The serologic diagnosis of heartworm infection in dogs and cats. *Clin Tech Small Anim Pract* 1998;13:83–87.

Gortel K. Equine parasitic hypersensitivity. *Equine Pract* 1998;20:14–16.

de Graaf DC, Vanopdenbosch E, Ortega-Mora LM, Abbassi H, Peeters JE. A review of the importance of cryptosporidiosis in farm animals. *Int J Parasitol* 1999;29:1269–1287.

Gunnarsson LK, Möller LC, Einarsson AM, Zakrisson G, Hagman BGJ, Christensson DA, Uggla AH, Hedhammar AA. Clinical efficacy of milbemycin oxime in the treatment of nasal mite infection in dogs. *J Am Anim Hosp Assoc* 1999;35:81–84.

Harrell LW, Deardorff TL. Human nanophyetiasis: transmission by handling naturally infected coho salmon (*Oncorhynchus kisutch*). *J Infect Dis* 1990;161:146–148.

Hendrix CM. Helminthic infections of the feline small and large intestines: diagnosis and treatment. *Vet Med* 1995; 90:456–472.

Hendrix CM. Identifying and controlling helminths of the feline esophagus, stomach, and liver. *Vet Med* 1995; 90:473–476.

Hendrix CM. *Diagnostic Veterinary Parasitology.* 2nd ed. St. Louis: Mosby; 1998.

Herd RP. Cestode infections in cattle, sheep, goats, and swine. In: Howard JL, Smith RA, eds. *Current Veterinary Therapy 4: Food Animal Practice.* Philadelphia: W.B. Saunders; 1999: 560–561.

Herd RP. Trematode infections in cattle, sheep, and goats. In: Howard JL, Smith RA, eds. *Current Veterinary Therapy 4: Food Animal Practice.* Philadelphia: W.B. Saunders; 1999:557–560.

Herd RP, Zajac AM. Nematode infections in cattle, sheep, goats, and swine. In: Howard JL, Smith RA, eds. *Current Veterinary Therapy 4: Food Animal Practice.* Philadelphia: W.B. Saunders; 1999:545–557.

Hutchens DE, Paul AJ, DiPietro JA. Treatment and control of gastrointestinal parasites. *Vet Clin N Am: Equine Pract* 1999;15:561–573.

Johnson EH, Windsor JJ, Muirhead DE, King GJ, Al-Busaidy R. Confirmation of the prophylactic value of paromomycin in a natural outbreak of caprine cryptosporidiosis. *Vet Res Commun* 2000;24:63–67.

Johnson RC. Canine spirocercosis and associated esophageal sarcoma. *Compen Contin Educ Pract Vet* 1992;14:577–580.

Jordan ME, Courtney CH. Equine tapeworm. *Equine Pract* 1999;21:10–14.

Kassai T. *Veterinary Helminthology*. Oxford: Butterworth–Heinemann; 1999.

Kazacos KR. *Baylisascaris* larva migrans. *J Am Vet Med Assoc* 1989;195:894–903.

Kemmerer DW. Heartworm disease in the domestic ferret. In: Seward RL, ed. *Recent Advances in Heartworm Disease: Symposium '98*. Batavia, IL: American Heartworm Society; 1998:87–89.

Kennedy MJ. Prevalence of eyeworms (Nematoda: Thelazioidea) in beef cattle grazing different range pasture zones in Alberta, Canada. *J Parasitol* 1993;79:866–869.

Kennedy MJ. The effect of treating beef cattle on pasture with ivermectin on the prevalence and intensity of *Thelazia* spp. (Nematoda: Thelazioidea) in the vector, *Musca autumnalis* (Diptera: Muscidae). *J Parasitol* 1994;80:321–326.

Kennedy MJ, MacKinnon JD. Site segregation of *Thelazia skrjabini* and *Thelazia gulosa* (Nematoda: Thelazioidea) in the eyes of cattle. *J Parasitol* 1994;80:501–504.

Kennedy MJ, Phyllips FE. Efficacy of doramectin against eyeworms (*Thelazia* spp.) in naturally and experimentally infected cattle. *Vet Parasitol* 1993;49:61–66.

Kirkpatrick CE, Nelson GR. Ivermectin treatment of urinary capillariasis in a dog. *J Am Vet Med Assoc* 1987;191:701–702.

Kittel DR, Campero C, Van Hoosear KA, Rhyan JC, BonDurant RH. Comparison of diagnostic methods for detection of active infection with *Tritrichomonas foetus* in beef heifers. *J Am Vet Med Assoc* 1998;213:519–522.

Knight DH, Lok JB. Seasonality of heartworm infection and implications for chemoprophylaxis. *Clin Tech Small Anim Pract* 1998;13:77–82.

Kocan AA, Breshears M, Cummings C, Panciera RJ, Ewing SA, Barker RW. Naturally occurring hepatozoonosis in coyotes from Oklahoma. *J Wildl Dis* 1999;35:86–89.

Kocan AA, Cummings CA, Panciera RG, Mathew JS, Ewing SA, Barker RW. Naturally occurring and experimentally transmitted *Hepatozoon americanum* in coyotes from Oklahoma. *J Wildl Dis* 2000;36:149–153.

Kvasnicka WG, Hall MR, Hanks DR. Bovine trichomoniasis. In: Howard JL, Smith RA, eds. *Current Veterinary Therapy 4: Food Animal Practice.* Philadelphia: W.B. Saunders; 1999:420–425.

Leib MS, Zajac AM. Giardiasis in dogs and cats. *Vet Med* 1999;94:793–802.

Lemarie SL. Canine demodicosis. *Compen Contin Educ Pract Vet* 1996;18:354–368.

Lillehoj HS, Lillehoj EP. Avian coccidiosis. A review of acquired intestinal immunity and vaccination strategies. *Avian Dis* 2000;44:408–425.

Lindsay DS, Upton SJ, Owen DSS, Morgan UM, Mead JR, Blagburn BL. *Cryptosporidium andersoni* n. sp. (Apicomplexa: Cryptosporidiae) from cattle, *Bos taurus*. *J Eukaryot Microbiol* 2000;47:91–95.

Little SE. Adult tapeworms in horses: clinical significance. *Compen Contin Educ Pract Vet* 1999;21:356–360.

Lloyd JE. Flies, lice, and grubs. In: Howard JL, Smith RA, eds. *Current Veterinary Therapy 4: Food Animal Practice*. Philadelphia: W.B. Saunders; 1999:706–713.

Love S, Murphy D, Mellor D. Pathogenicity of cyathostome infection. *Vet Parasitol* 1999;85:113–122.

Lun Z-R, Gajadhar AA. A simple and rapid method for staining *Tritrichomonas foetus* and *Trichomonas vaginalis*. *J Vet Diagn Invest* 1999;11:471–474.

Lyons ET, Tolliver SC, Drudge JH. Historical perspective of cyathostomes: prevalence, treatment, and control programs. *Vet Parasitol* 1999;85:97–112.

Lyons ET, Tolliver SC, Collins SS, Drudge JH, Granstrom DE. Transmission of some species of internal parasites in horses born in 1993, 1994, and 1995 on the same pasture on a farm in central Kentucky. *Vet Parasitol* 1997;70:225–240.

McAllister MM, Dubey JP, Lindsay DS, Jolley WT, Wills RA, McGuire AM. Dogs are definitive hosts of *Neospora caninum*. *Int J Parasitol* 1998;28:1473–1478.

McCall JW. Dirofilariasis in the domestic ferret. *Clin Tech Small Anim Pract* 1998;13:109–112.

MacKay RJ. Equine protozoal myeloencephalitis. *Vet Clin N Am: Equine Pract* 1997;1:79–96.

McKenna PB. Anthelmintic resistance in cattle nematodes in New Zealand: is it increasing? *N Z Vet J* 1996;44:76.

McKenna PB. Comparative evaluation of two emigration/sedimentation techniques for the recovery of dictyocaulid and protostrongylid larvae from faeces. *Vet Parasitol* 1999; 80:345–351.

Madden A, Pinckney RD, Forrest LJ. Canine paragonimosis. *Vet Med* 1999;94:783–791.

Mansfield LS, Schad GA. Ivermectin treatment of naturally acquired and experimentally induced *Strongyloides stercoralis* infections in dogs. *J Am Vet Med Assoc* 1992; 201:726–730.

Markovics A, Medinski B. Improved diagnosis of low intensity *Spirocerca lupi* infection by the sugar flotation method. *J Vet Diagn Invest* 1996;8:400–401.

Marks SL, Moore MP, Rishniw M. *Pneumonyssoides caninum*: the canine nasal mite. *Compen Contin Educ Pract Vet* 1994;16: 577–582.

Marsh AE, Barr BC, Packham AE, Conrad PA. Description of a new *Neospora* species (Protozoa: Apicomplexa: Sarcocystidae). *J Parasitol* 1998;84:983–991.

Mathew JS, Ewing SA, Panciera RJ, Woods JP. Experimental transmission of *Hepatozoon americanum* Vincent-Johnson et al., 1997 to dogs by the Gulf Coast tick, *Amblyomma maculatum* Koch. *Vet Parasitol* 1998;80:1–14.

Melhorn H, Schein E. Redescription of *Babesia equi* Laveran, 1901 as *Theileria equi* Melhorn, Schein 1998. *Parasitol Res* 1998;84:467–475.

Mense MG, Gardiner CH, Moeller RB, Partridge HL, Wilson S. Chronic emesis caused by a nematode-induced gastric nodule in a cat. *J Am Vet Med Assoc* 1992;201:597–598.

van Metre DC, Tyler JW, Stehman SM. Diagnosis of enteric disease in small ruminants. *Vet Clin N Am: Food Anim Pract* 2000;16:87–115.

Miller MM, Sweeney CR, Russell GE, Sheetz RM, Morrow JK. Effects of blood contamination of cerebrospinal fluid on Western blot analysis for detection of antibodies against *Sarcocystis neurona* and on albumin quotient and immunoglobulin G index in horses. *J Am Vet Med Assoc* 1999;215:67–71.

Miller MW. Canine heartworm disease. *Clin Tech Small Anim Pract* 1998;13:113–118.

Miller PE, Campbell BG. Subconjunctival cyst associated with *Thelazia gulosa* in a calf. *J Am Vet Med Assoc* 1992; 201:1058–1060.

Miller Jr. WH, Scott DW, Wellington JR, Panić R. Clinical efficacy of milbemycin oxime in the treatment of generalized demodicosis in adult dogs. *J Am Vet Med Assoc* 1993; 203:1426–1429.

Munoz E, Castella J, Gutierrez JF. In vivo and in vitro sensitivity of *Trichomonas gallinae* to some nitroimidazole drugs. *Vet Parasitol* 1998;78:239–246.

Olson ME, McAllister TA, Deselliers L, Morck DW, Cheng K-J, Buret AG, Ceri H. Effects of giardiasis on production in a domestic ruminant (lamb) model. *Am J Vet Res* 1995;56:1470–1474.

Ortega-Mora LM, Requejo-Fernandez JA, Pilar-Izquierdo M, Pereira-Bueno J. Role of adult sheep in transmission of infection by *Cryptosporidium parvum* to lambs: confirmation of periparturient rise. *Int J Parasitol* 1999;29:1261–1268.

Panciera RJ, Ewing SA, Mathew JS, Lehenbauer TW, Cummings CA, Woods JP. Canine hepatozoonosis: comparison of lesions and parasites in skeletal muscle of dogs experimentally or naturally infected with *Hepatozoon americanum.* *Vet Parasitol* 1999;82:261–272.

Panciera RJ, Ewing SA, Mathew JS, Cummings CA, Kocan AA, Breshears MA, Fox JC. Observations on tissue stages of *Hepatozoon americanum* in 19 naturally infected dogs. *Vet Parasitol* 1998;78:265–276.

Paradis M. Ivermectin in small animal dermatology. Part II. Extralabel applications. *Compen Contin Edu Pract Vet* 1998;20:459–469.

Parker S, Campbell J, Ribble C, Gajadhar A. Comparison of two sampling tools for diagnosis of *Tritrichomonas foetus* in bulls and clinical interpretation of culture results. *J Am Vet Med Assoc* 1999;215:231–235.

Perris EE. Parasitic dermatoses that cause pruritus in horses. *Vet Clin N Am: Equine Pract* 1995;11:11–28.

Proudman CJ, Trees AJ. Tapeworms as a cause of intestinal disease in horses. *Parasitol Today* 1999;56:156–159.

Proudman CJ, French NP, Trees AJ. Tapeworm infection is a significant risk factor for spasmodic colic and ileal impaction colic in the horse. *Equine Vet J* 1998;30:194–199.

Rae DO, Chenoweth PJ, Genho PC, McIntosh AD, Crosby CE, Moore SA. Prevalence of *Tritrichomonas fetus* in a bull population and effect on production in a large cow-calf enterprise. *J Am Vet Med Assoc* 1999;214:1051–1055.

Rallis T, Vlemmas J. Gastroesophageal intussusception in an adult dog. *Canine Pract* 1995;20:7–11.

Rausch RL. Life cycle patterns and geographic distribution of *Echinococcus* species. In: Thompson RCA, Lymbery AJ, eds. *Echinococcus and Hydatid Disease.* Wallingford, CT: CAB International; 1999:89–134.

Ridley RK. Parasites of the respiratory system. In: Howard JL, Smith RA, eds. *Current Veterinary Therapy 4: Food Animal Practice.* Philadelphia: W.B. Saunders; 1999:460–462.

Robertson-Plouch CK, Dillon AR, Brawner Jr. WR, Guerrero J. Prevalence of feline heartworm infections among cats with respiratory and gastrointestinal signs: results of a multi-center study. *Vet Ther: Res Appl Vet Med* 2000;1:88–95.

Ruest N, Couture Y, Faubert GM, Girard C. Morphological changes in the jejunum of calves naturally infected with *Giardia* spp. and *Cryptosporidium* spp. *Vet Parasitol* 1997; 69:177–186.

Sanderson MW, Gay JM, Baszler TV. *Neospora caninum* sero-prevalence and associated risk factors in beef cattle in the northwestern United States. *Vet Parasitol* 2000;90:15–24.

Schantz PM, Chai J, Craig PS, Eckert J, Jenkins DJ, Macpherson CNL, Thakur A. Epidemiology and control of hydatid disease. In: Thompson RCA, Lymbery AJ, eds. *Echinococcus and Hydatid Disease.* Wallingford, CT: CAB International; 1999:233–331.

Schwartz RD, Donoghue AR, Baggs RB, Clark T, Partington C. Evaluation of the safety of fenbendazole in cats. *Am J Vet Res* 2000;61:330–333.

Shorter N, Werninghaus K, Mooney D, Graham A. Furuncular cuterebrid myiasis. *J Ped Surg* 1997;32:1511–1513.

Sloss MW, Kemp RL, Zajac AM. *Veterinary Clinical Parasitology.* 6th ed. Ames: Iowa State University Press; 1994.

Soulsby EJL. *Helminths, Arthropods and Protozoa of Domesticated Animals.* 7th ed. London: Baillière Tindall; 1982.

Speer CA. Coccidiosis. In: Howard JL, Smith RA, eds. *Current Veterinary Therapy 4: Food Animal Practice.* Philadelphia: W.B. Saunders; 1999:411–420.

Thompson RCA. Biology and systematics of *Echinococcus.* In: Thompson RCA, Lymbery AJ, eds. *Echinococcus and Hydatid Disease.* Wallingford, CT: CAB International; 1999:1–50.

Thompson RCA, Hopkins RM, Homan WL. Nomenclature and genetic groupings of *Giardia* infecting mammals. *Parasitol Today* 2000;16:210–213.

Thrumond MC, Hietala SD. *Neospora caninum* infection and abortion in cattle. In: Howard JL, Smith RA, eds. *Current Veterinary Therapy 4: Food Animal Practice.* Philadelphia: W.B. Saunders; 1999:425–431.

Tranas J, Heinzen RA, Weiss LM, McAllister MM. Serological evidence of human infection with the protozoan *Neospora caninum. Clin Diagn Lab Immunol* 1999;6:765–767.

Trees AJ. Parasitic diseases. In: Jordan FTW, Pattison M, eds. *Poultry Diseases.* 4th ed. London: W.B. Saunders; 1996:261–289.

Trees AJ, Davison HC, Innes EA, Wastling JM. Towards evaluating the economic impact of bovine neosporosis. *Int J Parasitol* 1999;29:1195–1200.

Vincent-Johnson N, Macintire DK, Baneth G. Canine hepato-zoonosis: pathophysiology, diagnosis, and treatment. *Compen Contin Educ Pract Vet* 1997;19:51–65.

Vincent-Johnson NA, Macintire DK, Lindsay DS, Lenz SD, Baneth G, Shkap V. A new *Hepatozoon* species from dogs: description of the causative agent of canine hepatozoonosis in North America. *J Parasitol* 1997;83:1165–1172.

Williamson RMC, Beveridge I, Gasser RB. Coprological methods for the diagnosis of *Anoplocephala perfoliata* infection of the horse. *Aust Vet J* 1998;76:618–621.

de Wit JJ. Mortality of rheas caused by a *Synchamus trachea* infection. *Vet Quart* 1995;17:39–40.

Xiao L. *Giardia* infection in farm animals. *Parasitol Today* 1994;11:436–438.

Index

Page numbers followed by "t" indicate tables; page numbers followed by "f" indicate figures.